THE INSULIN RESISTANCE RESET COOKBOOK FOR BEGINNERS

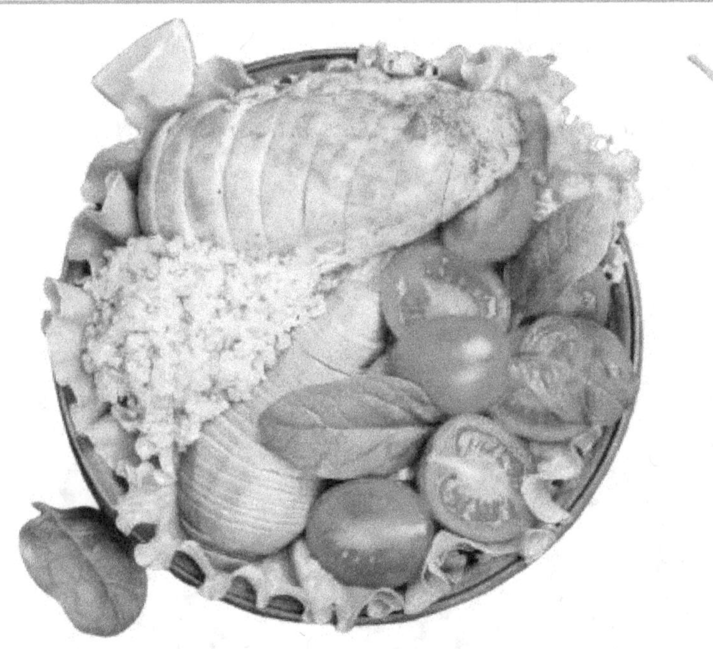

No Stress Tasty Recipes to Manage PCOS, Weight Loss, Stop Pre-Diabetes and Boost Healthy Well-Being

Joan G. Milone

Copyright © 2024 by Joan G. Milone

All rights reserved.

This book is written as a source of information only. The information contained in this book is provided in good faith and is believed to be accurate and reliable as of the date of publication. The author does not assume any responsibility for any errors or omissions that may appear.

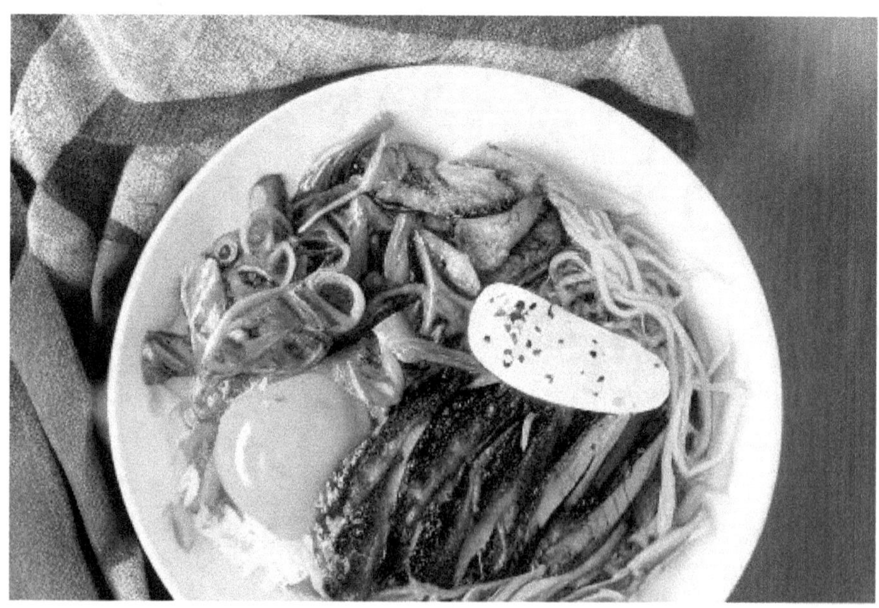

Table of Contents

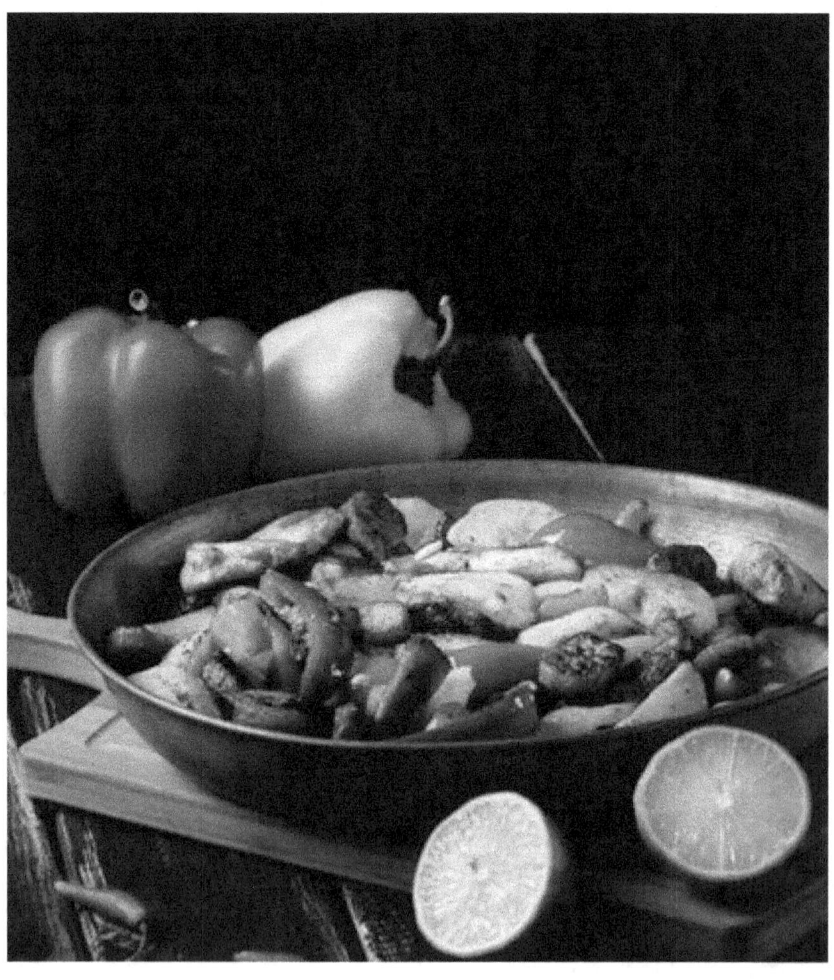

Introduction

Welcome to our journey together in this cookbook, where we explore a new way of eating tailored to managing insulin resistance. If you've ever felt overwhelmed or isolated by your dietary needs, this book is for you. We're going to transform how you think about food, turning dietary restrictions into a celebration of delicious, healthful eating.

I understand how challenging it can be to navigate a condition that requires such careful attention to what you eat. That's why every recipe in this book is designed not only to stabilize your blood sugar but also to delight your palate. From vibrant smoothies to start your day, to nourishing stews that comfort you in the evening, each dish is a step toward better health.

This cookbook is more than a collection of recipes—it's a companion in your culinary journey. It's about creating joyous meals that you can look forward to cooking and eating. Managing insulin resistance isn't just about avoiding certain foods; it's about embracing a lifestyle that enhances your overall wellbeing.

As we move through each section, from breakfasts to desserts, I'll share tips and insights that make cooking easier and more enjoyable. These recipes are designed to bring excitement back to your table and to help you feel empowered in your dietary choices.

Join me as we embark on this adventure together. With each page turned and every recipe tried, you'll gain confidence in the kitchen. Here's to delicious meals that make you feel great and keep you healthy. Let's cook up joy and wellness, one dish at a time. Welcome to a new way of cooking, a new way of eating, and a new way of living.

The Power of Food: Transforming Your Health

Food is more than just food; it is an essential part of our lives, influencing our health, mood, and well-being. This book focuses on the important role food plays in reducing insulin resistance and improving your health. It is here to demonstrate that with each dish, you can improve your body's health.

Managing insulin resistance can be difficult, but the appropriate foods can make the process much easier. The recipes and instructions provided here will teach you how each component and meal can help regulate blood sugar levels, reduce inflammation, and improve your overall health.

The idea is straightforward: consume foods that nourish and support your body's needs while relishing the flavors and pleasures of well-prepared meals. The recipes in this book emphasize nutritious, nutrient-dense ingredients that enhance overall health. Incorporating complex carbohydrates, lean proteins, and healthy fats will not only help you control your insulin resistance more efficiently but will also lead to increased energy and vitality.

Furthermore, this book contains more than just recipes. It is a guide to learning how different foods affect your blood sugar, how to prepare meals that improve your metabolic health, and how to make lifestyle decisions that promote long-term well-being.

Every part, from appetizers to sweets, is an invitation to discover how delicious and healthy meals can coexist. Whether you're new to regulating your diet for health reasons or want to broaden your culinary horizons, this book will inspire you and demonstrate the healing power of food.

Embrace this journey as an opportunity to improve your health through the foods you make and consume. Allow food to help you live a more vibrant, healthier life. Here's to a new relationship with food—one that empowers, nourishes, and heals.

How to Use This Cookbook

1. Familiarize Yourself with the Basics:

Start by reading the introduction and any guides included in the book, such as the substitution guide or the section on navigating social situations. Understanding these basics will help you make the most of the recipes and tips provided, ensuring that you're well-prepared to start your cooking journey.

2. Plan Your Meals:

Use the meal planning and prep guide to start organizing your meals for the week. This section will help you understand how to balance your meals effectively, ensuring you get a good mix of proteins, carbohydrates, and fats. Plan around your schedule and dietary needs to make your meal preparation seamless and stress-free.

3. Shop Effectively:

Refer to the comprehensive shopping list provided to gather all the ingredients you'll need. Organize your shopping list by category to save time in the grocery store. Consider purchasing some pantry staples in bulk, which can save money and reduce the frequency of your shopping trips.

4. Cook with Confidence:

Choose a recipe that appeals to you and fits your meal plan. Each recipe comes with detailed instructions and nutritional information. Start with simpler recipes to build your confidence if you're new to the kitchen, and then progress to more complex dishes as you become more comfortable.

5. **Reflect and Adjust:**

After preparing and enjoying your meals, take some time to reflect on the experience. What did you enjoy? What might you change next time? Use this feedback to adjust your future meal plans and recipes. Remember, this cookbook is not just a guide but a tool for learning and adapting to your tastes and nutritional needs.

By following these steps, you'll be able to make full use of the cookbook and incorporate its recipes into a healthy, enjoyable eating routine tailored to managing insulin resistance. Enjoy the process of exploring new flavors and creating meals that nourish both your body and spirit.

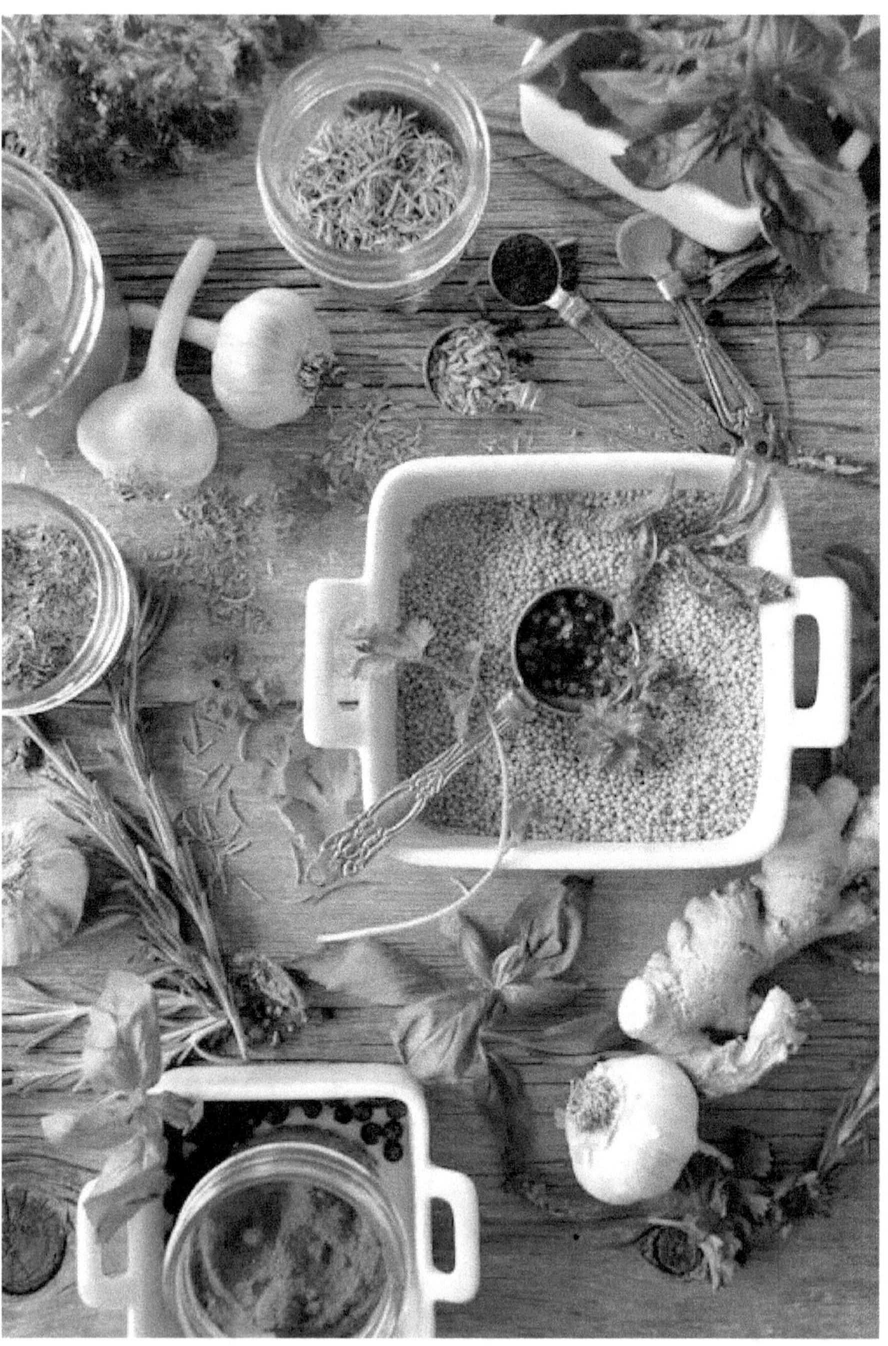

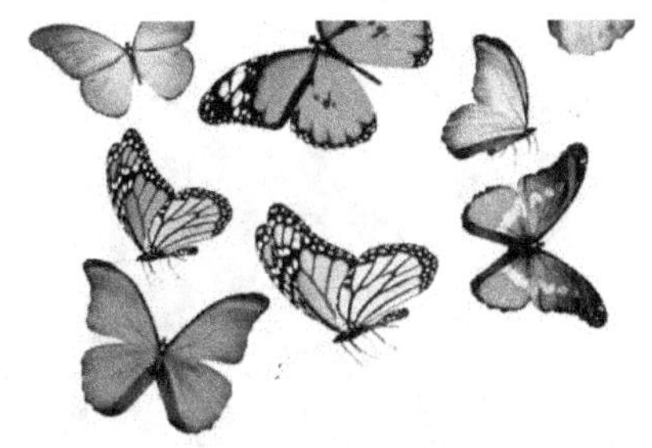

Part 1: The Basics

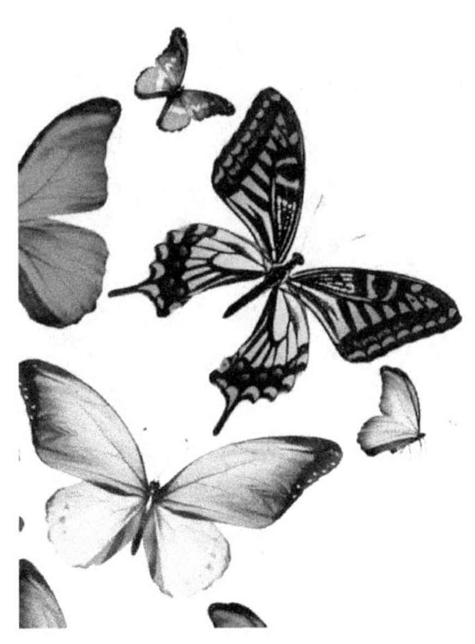

Beginner's Guide to Insulin-Resistant Cooking

If you're starting to manage insulin resistance through nutrition, you should know how to prepare meals that assist you in maintaining stable blood sugar levels. This guide is intended to provide you with the fundamental knowledge and practical advice you need to cook confidently and enjoyably in your kitchen.

Insulin resistance occurs when cells fail to respond to insulin, resulting in elevated blood sugar levels and type 2 diabetes. Your diet can help manage these effects by keeping blood sugar levels constant.

Foods to Focus On:

Focus on foods with low to moderate glycemic index (GI), which have a slower effect on blood sugar levels. Fill your plate with fiber-rich veggies, entire grains, lean proteins, and healthy fats. Some excellent choices include:

Vegetables: Opt for leafy greens, broccoli, cauliflower, and other non-starchy alternatives.

Whole Grains: Look for quinoa, oats, and barley.

Proteins: Choose chicken, turkey, fish, tofu, and lentils.

Fats: Include healthy fats such as avocados, nuts, seeds, and olive oil.

Cooking Procedures:

Use procedures that preserve nutritional content and reduce additional fats and sugars. Steaming, baking, grilling, and stir-frying are the finest options. When sautéing, use healthy oils such as olive oil sparingly.

Balancing Meals:

To maintain stable blood glucose levels, balance your meals with a variety of carbohydrates, proteins, and fats. A lunch, for example, could include lean protein, complete grains, and plenty of veggies, resulting in a fulfilling and balanced diet.

Mindful Eating:

To prevent blood sugar spikes, practice mindful eating by eating at regular intervals and limiting portion sizes. Skipping meals can lead to future overeating and make blood sugar regulation more difficult.

By following these instructions, you can better manage your insulin resistance, enhance your health, and enjoy a wide range of delicious meals.

Kitchen Essentials for Healthy Cooking

Equipping your kitchen with the right tools can make all the difference in preparing healthy and delicious meals efficiently. Here's a guide to the essential kitchen gadgets and cookware that will help you whip up the nutritious recipes from our cookbook:

1. Quality Knives: A sharp chef's knife and a paring knife are crucial for efficient chopping, slicing, and dicing of vegetables, meats, and fruits. Investing in good-quality knives can save you time and improve the precision of your cuts.

2. Cutting Boards: Have at least two cutting boards to avoid cross-contamination—one for fresh produce and the other for raw meats. Bamboo and plastic are great options as they are durable and easy to clean.

3. Blenders and Food Processors: A high-powered blender is perfect for making smoothies, soups, and sauces. A food processor is ideal for more labor-intensive tasks like chopping vegetables, grinding nuts and seeds, or making doughs and batters.

4. Measuring Cups and Spoons: Accurate measurements are important for following recipes correctly, especially when you are watching your intake of certain ingredients. Stainless steel measuring tools are recommended for their longevity and ease of cleaning.

5. Non-Stick Skillet and Pots: A good set of non-stick cookware will minimize the amount of oil needed for cooking, helping to keep your meals lower in fat. Look for PFOA-free non-stick surfaces for safety.

6. Mixing Bowls: A set of mixing bowls in various sizes is useful for preparing ingredients and mixing them. Opt for bowls that are microwave-safe to make reheating ingredients easier.

7. Baking Sheets and Silicone Mats: For roasting vegetables and baking, baking sheets are indispensable. Pair them with silicone mats or parchment paper to prevent sticking without added oils.

8. Steamer Basket: Steaming is a healthy way to cook vegetables, fish, and even chicken, preserving more nutrients than many other cooking methods. A steamer basket can be used with your existing pots.

9. Spatulas and Wooden Spoons: Silicone spatulas are great for scraping bowls without scratching surfaces, and wooden spoons are perfect for stirring dishes without conducting heat.

10. Digital Food Scale: A food scale is essential for those who need precise ingredient measurements, which can be crucial for maintaining dietary requirements.

11. Slow Cooker or Pressure Cooker: These appliances are excellent for making stews, soups, and braised dishes with minimal effort. They allow for better infusion of flavors and can be very energy efficient.

Having these tools at your disposal will not only enhance your cooking experience but also help ensure that you can easily prepare healthy meals. Each tool serves a purpose to help you manage your diet effectively, cook with less fat, and enjoy a variety of cooking techniques that keep your meals interesting and nutritious.

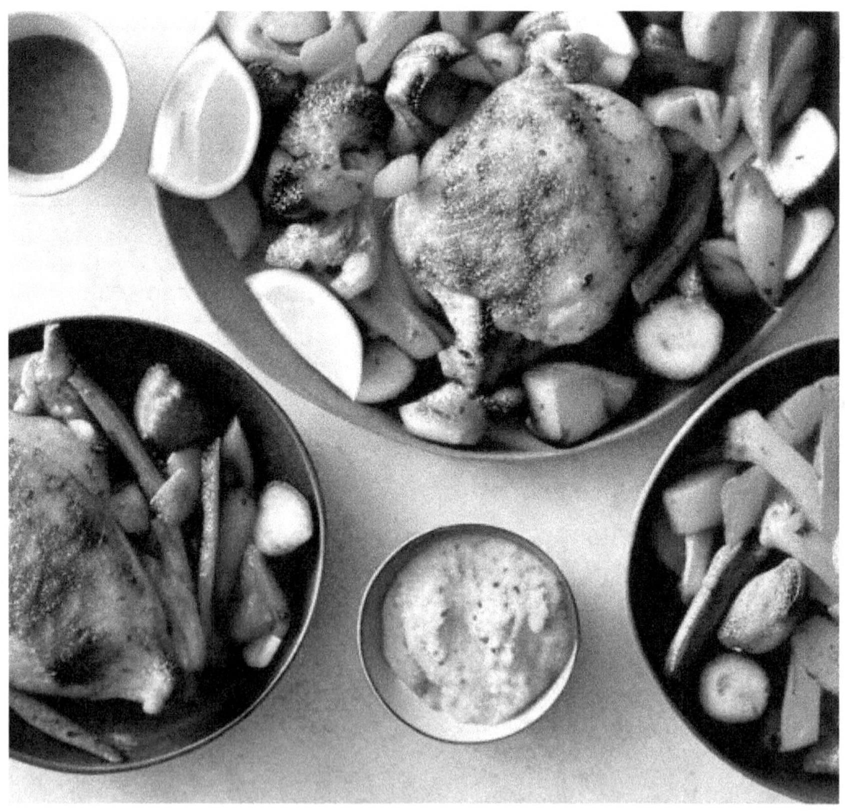

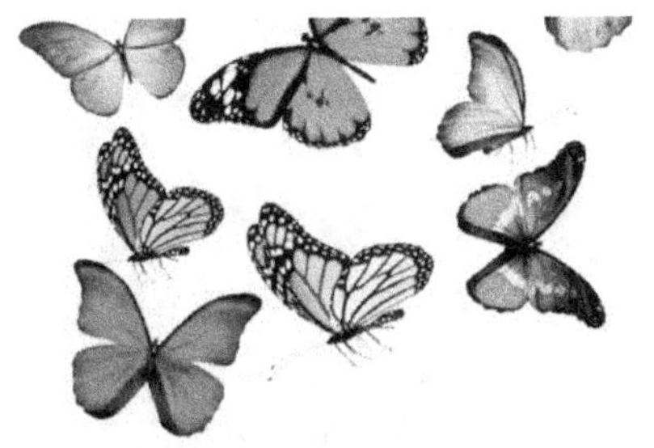

Part 2: Quick and Easy Recipes

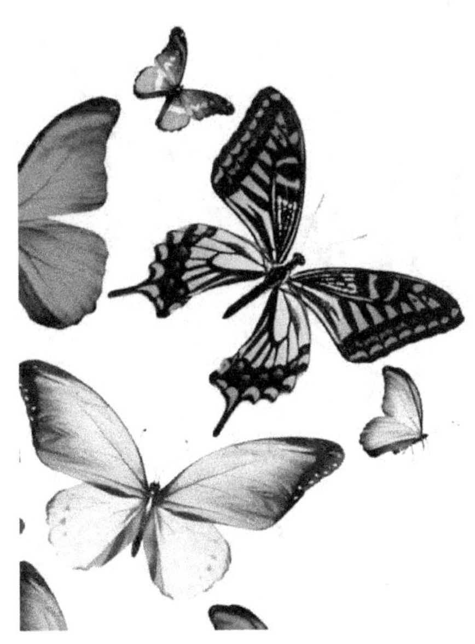

Breakfast and Smoothies

Start your day with our breakfast and smoothie recipes, which are meant to provide energy and maintain blood sugar balance. Quick, nutritious, and delicious, they're ideal for controlling insulin resistance and feeding your day without causing a sugar spike. Enjoy a range of flavors and minerals that promote healthy eating throughout the day.

Almond and Berry Smoothie

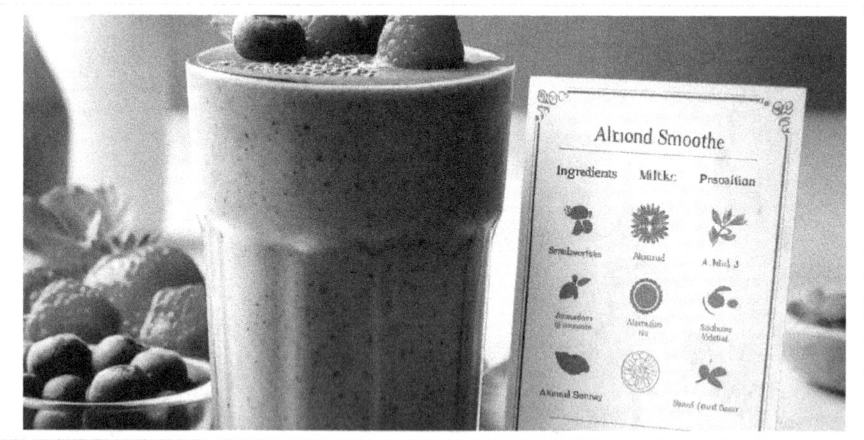

Ingredients:

- 1 cup mixed berries (strawberries, blueberries, raspberries)
- 1 banana
- 2 tablespoons almonds
- 1 cup almond milk

- 1 tablespoon chia seeds

Preparation:

1. Blend mixed berries, banana, almonds, and almond milk until smooth.
2. Pour into a glass and garnish with chia seeds.

Nutritional Values: (per serving)

- Calories: 280
- Protein: 8g
- Fat: 9g

- Carbohydrates: 44g
- Fiber: 10g

Cooking Time: 5 minutes

Serves: 2

Rating: ★★★★☆

Chia Seed Pudding

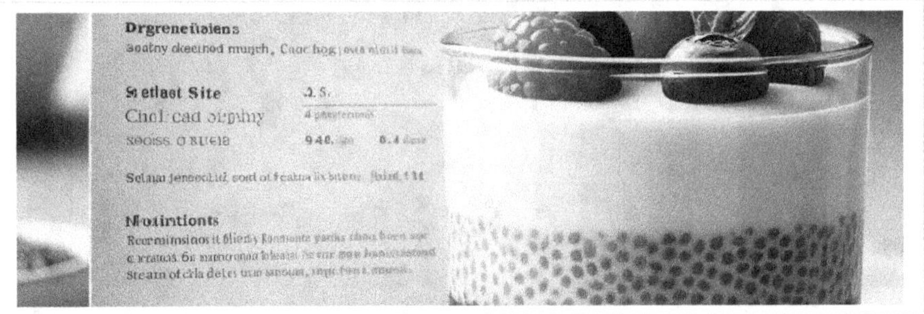

Ingredients:

- 1/4 cup chia seeds
- 1 cup almond milk
- 1 tablespoon maple syrup

- 1/2 teaspoon vanilla extract
- Fresh berries for topping

Preparation:

1. Mix chia seeds, almond milk, maple syrup, and vanilla extract in a bowl.
2. Refrigerate for at least 4 hours or overnight until it thickens.
3. Serve topped with fresh berries.

Nutritional Values: (per serving)

- Calories: 150
- Protein: 4g
- Fat: 7g
- Carbohydrates: 18g
- Fiber: 9g

Cooking Time: 5 minutes + chilling time

Serves: 2

Rating: ★★★★☆

Avocado Toast with Poached Egg

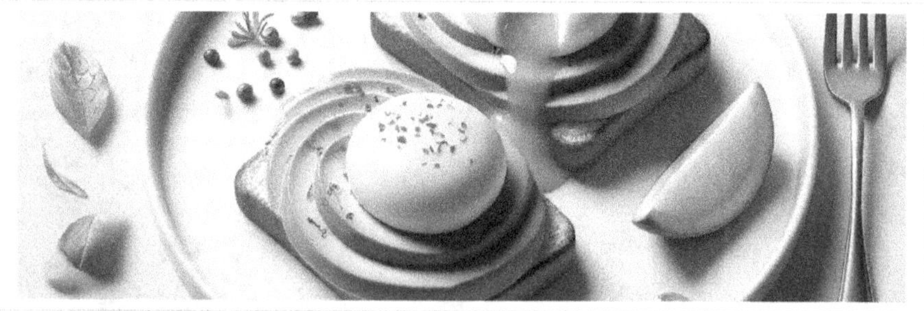

Ingredients:

- 1 ripe avocado
- 2 eggs
- 2 slices of whole-grain bread
- Salt and pepper to taste

- Chili flakes (optional)

Preparation:

1. Poach eggs to desired doneness in simmering water.
2. Toast bread slices until golden.
3. Mash avocado and spread evenly on toast.
4. Top each toast with a poached egg.
5. Season with salt, pepper, and chili flakes.

Nutritional Values: (per serving)

- Calories: 350
- Protein: 14g
- Fat: 25g

- Carbohydrates: 26g
- Fiber: 7g

Cooking Time: 15 minutes

Serves: 2

Rating: ★★★★★

Spinach and Feta Omelet

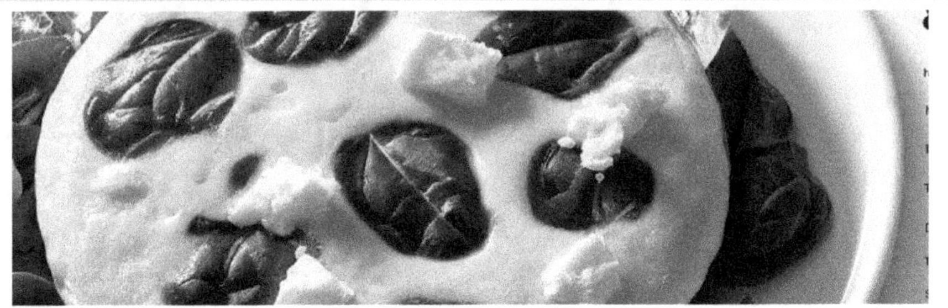

Ingredients:

- 2 eggs

- 1/2 cup fresh spinach, chopped
- 1/4 cup feta cheese, crumbled
- Salt and pepper to taste
- 1 tablespoon olive oil

Preparation:

1. Beat the eggs in a bowl and season with salt and pepper.
2. Heat olive oil in a skillet over medium heat.
3. Add the spinach and sauté until wilted.
4. Pour the eggs over the spinach and cook until the edges start to set.
5. Sprinkle feta cheese over the omelet.
6. Fold the omelet in half and cook until golden brown on both sides.

Nutritional Values: (per serving)

- Calories: 300
- Protein: 20g
- Fat: 23g
- Carbohydrates: 2g
- Fiber: 1g

Cooking Time: 10 minutes

Serves: 1

Rating: ★★★★★

Quinoa Breakfast Bowl

Ingredients:

- 1 cup cooked quinoa
- 1 soft-boiled egg
- 1/2 avocado, sliced
- 1/4 cup fresh berries (strawberries, blueberries)
- 1 tablespoon chia seeds
- 2 tablespoons nuts (almonds, walnuts)

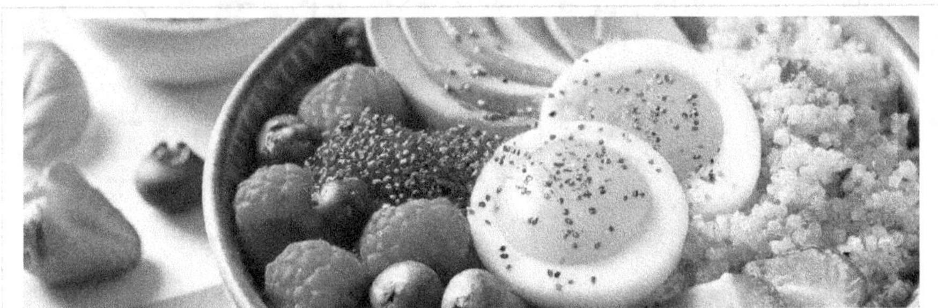

Preparation:

1. Prepare quinoa according to package instructions.
2. Soft-boil the egg to your liking.
3. Slice the avocado and rinse the berries.
4. In a bowl, layer the cooked quinoa, soft-boiled egg, avocado slices, and berries.
5. Sprinkle chia seeds and nuts on top.

Nutritional Values: (per serving)

- Calories: 450
- Protein: 15g
- Fat: 25g
- Carbohydrates: 45g
- Fiber: 10g

Cooking Time: 20 minutes

Serves: 1

Rating: ★★★★☆

Green Detox Smoothie

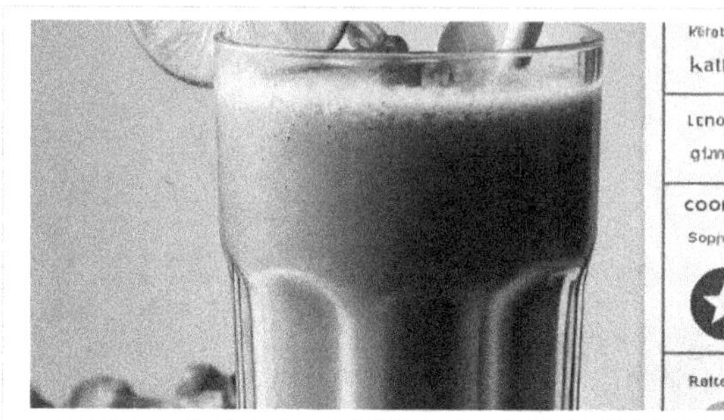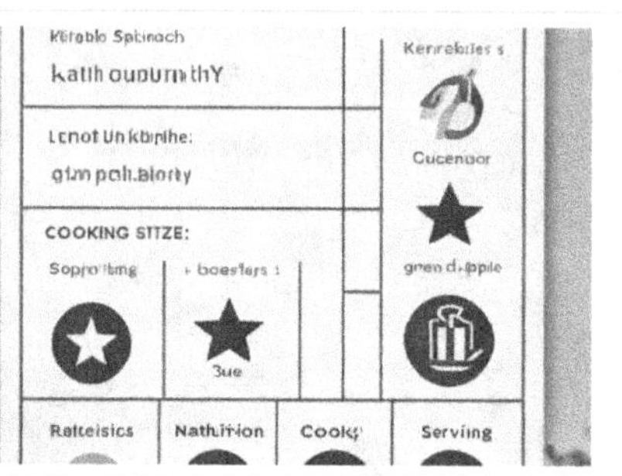

Ingredients:

- 1 cup spinach
- 1 cup kale, chopped
- 1/2 cucumber
- 1 green apple, cored and sliced
- Juice of 1 lemon
- 1 inch ginger, peeled

Preparation:

1. Add all ingredients to a blender.
2. Blend until smooth.
3. Serve immediately, garnished with a slice of lime.

Nutritional Values: (per serving)

- Calories: 120
- Protein: 3g
- Fat: 0.5g
- Carbohydrates: 30g
- Fiber: 5g

Cooking Time: 5 minutes

Serves: 1　　　　　　　　**Rating:** ★★★★☆

Protein Pancakes

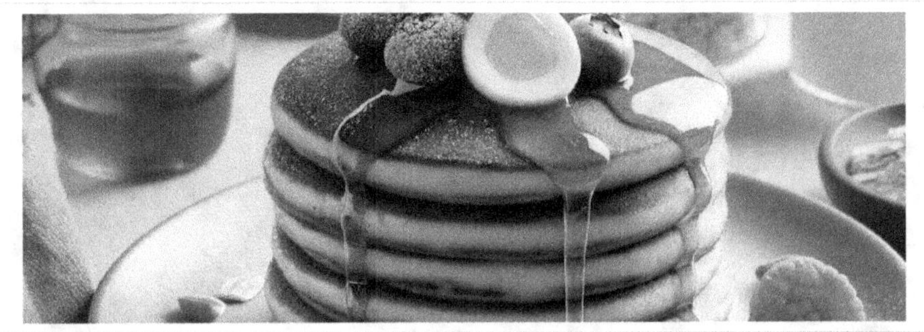

Ingredients:

- 1 scoop protein powder
- 1/2 cup oats
- 1 egg
- 1 banana
- 1/2 cup almond milk

Preparation:

1. Blend oats into a flour.
2. Mix all ingredients in a blender until smooth.
3. Cook on a non-stick skillet over medium heat until bubbles form, then flip.
4. Serve with honey and fresh berries.

Nutritional Values: (per serving)

- Calories: 320
- Protein: 22g
- Fat: 5g
- Carbohydrates: 50g
- Fiber: 6g

Cooking Time: 15 minutes

Serves: 2   **Rating:** ★★★★☆

Overnight Oats with Nuts

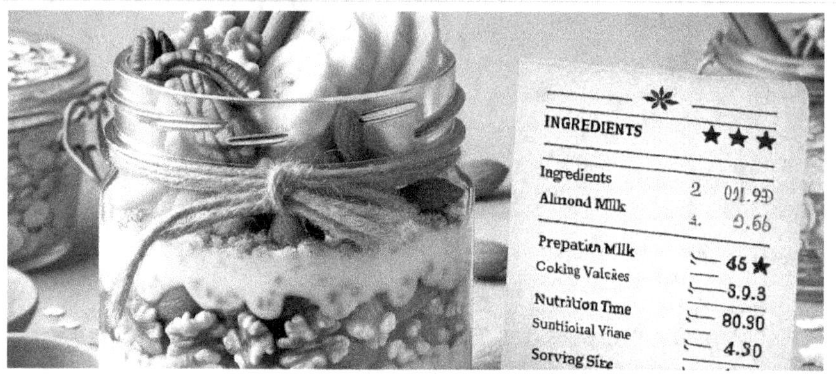

Ingredients:

- 1/2 cup rolled oats
- 3/4 cup almond milk
- 1 tablespoon mixed nuts (almonds, walnuts, pecans), chopped
- 1/2 banana, sliced
- 1 teaspoon honey
- A pinch of cinnamon

Preparation:

1. In a jar, combine oats and almond milk.
2. Add chopped nuts and a pinch of cinnamon. Stir to mix.
3. Seal the jar and refrigerate overnight.
4. Top with banana slices and drizzle with honey before serving.

Nutritional Values: (per serving)

- Calories: 350
- Protein: 10g
- Fat: 15g
- Carbohydrates: 45g
- Fiber: 7g

Cooking Time: 8 hours (overnight)

Serves: 1

Rating: ★★★★☆

Breakfast Tacos with Cauliflower Tortilla

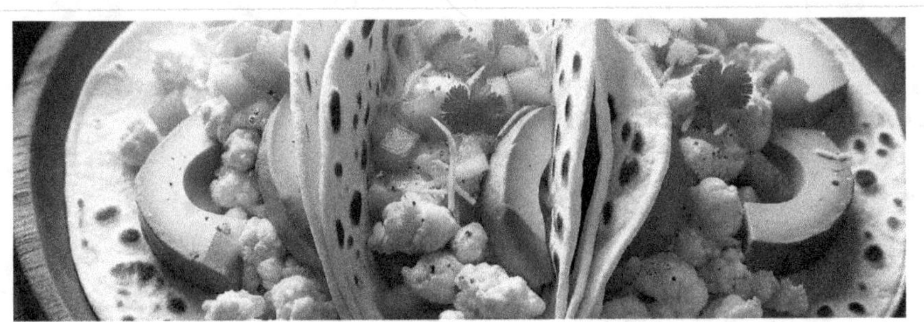

Ingredients:

- 2 cauliflower tortillas
- 4 eggs, scrambled
- 1 avocado, sliced
- 1/2 cup diced tomatoes
- 1/4 cup shredded cheese
- Fresh cilantro for garnish
- Salsa for serving

Preparation:

1. Prepare the cauliflower tortillas according to your favorite recipe.
2. Scramble the eggs in a skillet over medium heat.

3. Warm the tortillas, then fill each with scrambled eggs, avocado slices, and diced tomatoes.

4. Sprinkle shredded cheese on top.

5. Garnish with fresh cilantro and serve with salsa on the side.

Nutritional Values: (per serving)

- Calories: 400
- Protein: 20g
- Fat: 30g

- Carbohydrates: 15g
- Fiber: 7g

Cooking Time: 30 minutes

Serves: 2

Rating: ★★★★☆

Yogurt and Granola Parfait

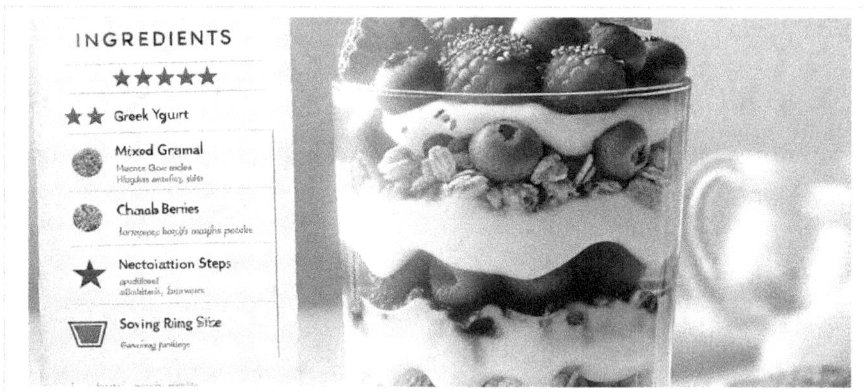

Ingredients:

- 1 cup Greek yogurt
- 1/2 cup granola

- 1/2 cup mixed berries (strawberries, blueberries, raspberries)

- 1 tablespoon chia seeds
- Mint leaves for garnish

Preparation:

1. In a clear glass, layer 1/2 cup of Greek yogurt.
2. Add a layer of 1/4 cup granola.
3. Add a layer of 1/4 cup mixed berries.
4. Repeat the layers.
5. Top with chia seeds and a mint leaf.

Nutritional Values: (per serving)

- Calories: 350
- Protein: 20g
- Fat: 10g
- Carbohydrates: 45g
- Fiber: 5g

Cooking Time: 5 minutes

Serves: 1

Rating: ★★★★★

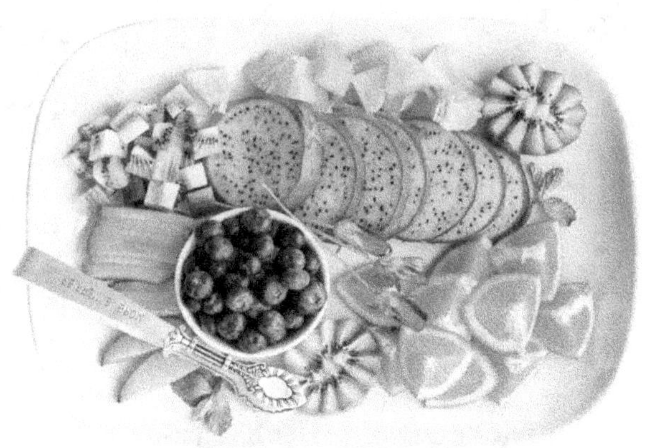

Lunch

Lunchtime in our cookbook is about more than simply eating; it's an opportunity to nurture your body, reset your mind, and keep your energy levels high throughout the afternoon. These recipes are designed with insulin resistance in mind, so you can enjoy balanced, delicious meals that help you achieve your health objectives. From vivid salads and hearty sandwiches to fulfilling bowls, each item is intended to be simple to prepare, easily portable for hectic schedules, and, most importantly, delicious to eat. Dive into these lunch options that will keep you full, focused, and on track with your nutritional needs.

Chickpea and Avocado Salad

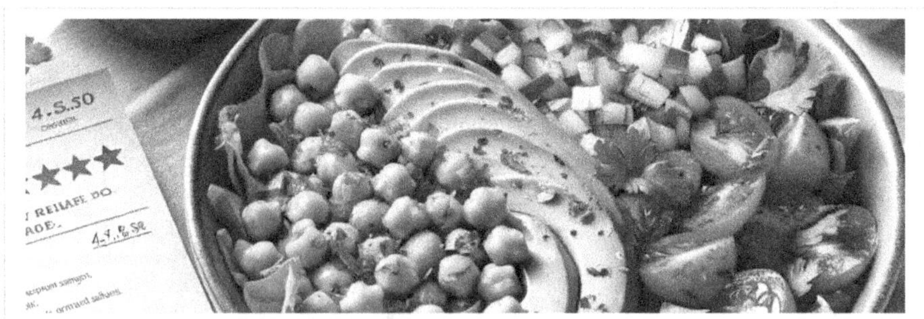

Ingredients:

- 1 can (15 oz) chickpeas, drained and rinsed

- 1 ripe avocado, cubed

- 1 cup fresh greens (spinach or arugula)
- 1/2 cup diced tomatoes
- 1/4 cup diced red onion
- For the dressing:
  - o 2 tablespoons olive oil
  - o Juice of 1 lemon
  - o Salt and pepper to taste
- Fresh cilantro for garnish

Preparation:

1. In a large bowl, combine chickpeas, avocado, greens, tomatoes, and red onion.
2. In a small bowl, whisk together olive oil, lemon juice, salt, and pepper.
3. Pour the dressing over the salad and toss gently to combine.
4. Garnish with fresh cilantro before serving.

Nutritional Values: (per serving)

- Calories: 300
- Protein: 10g
- Fat: 20g
- Carbohydrates: 27g
- Fiber: 10g

Cooking Time: 10 minutes

Serves: 2

Rating: ★★★★☆

Turkey and Spinach Wrap

Ingredients:

- 2 whole wheat tortillas
- 4 slices of turkey breast
- 1 cup fresh spinach
- 1/2 cup shredded carrots
- 1 avocado, sliced
- Light yogurt dressing for dipping

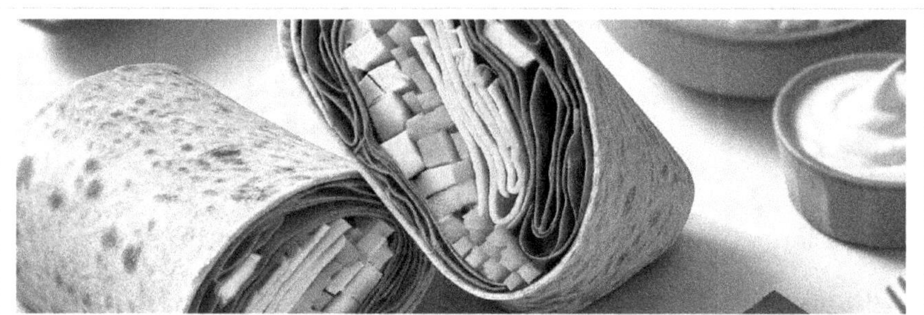

Preparation:

1. Lay out the tortillas on a flat surface.
2. Distribute the turkey slices evenly over each tortilla.
3. Add a layer of spinach, shredded carrots, and avocado slices on top of the turkey.
4. Roll the tortillas tightly around the fillings.
5. Cut each wrap in half and serve with a side of yogurt dressing.

Nutritional Values: (per serving)

- Calories: 350
- Protein: 25g
- Fat: 15g
- Carbohydrates: 35g
- Fiber: 6g

Cooking Time: 10 minutes

Serves: 2

Rating: ★★★★★

Quinoa and Black Bean Bowl

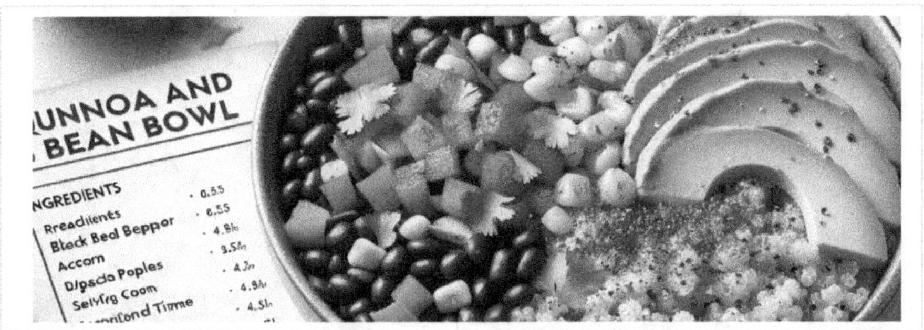

Ingredients:

- 1 cup cooked quinoa
- 1 can (15 oz) black beans, drained and rinsed
- 1 red bell pepper, diced
- 1/2 cup corn (fresh or frozen)
- 1 avocado, sliced
- Chopped cilantro for garnish
- Lime wedge for serving

Preparation:

1. Prepare quinoa according to package instructions.
2. In a bowl, layer the cooked quinoa as the base.
3. Top with black beans, diced red bell pepper, and corn.
4. Add avocado slices on top.
5. Garnish with chopped cilantro and serve with a lime wedge on the side.

Nutritional Values: (per serving)

- Calories: 400
- Protein: 14g

- Fat: 12g
- Carbohydrates: 64g

- Fiber: 15g

Cooking Time: 20 minutes

Serves: 2

Rating: ★★★★★

Grilled Vegetable Platter

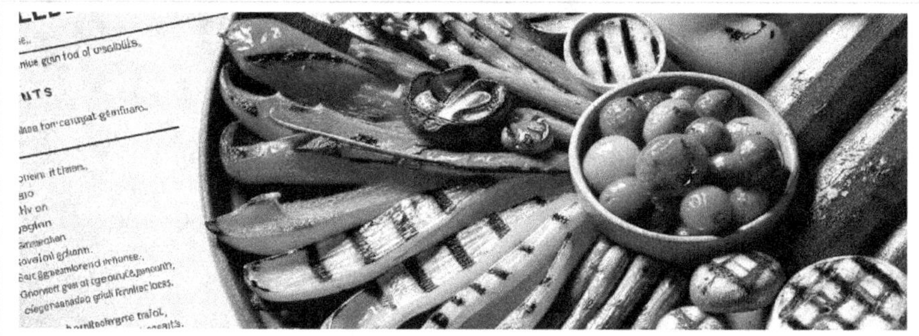

Ingredients:

- 1 zucchini, sliced
- 2 bell peppers (red and yellow), sliced
- 1 bunch asparagus, trimmed
- 1 cup mushrooms, whole

- 1 cup cherry tomatoes
- Olive oil for brushing
- Salt and pepper to taste
- Side of hummus
- Balsamic glaze for drizzling

Preparation:

1. Preheat grill to medium-high heat.
2. Brush vegetables with olive oil and season with salt and pepper.
3. Grill vegetables until tender and charred, turning occasionally.

4. Arrange grilled vegetables on a platter.

5. Serve with a side of hummus and drizzle with balsamic glaze.

Nutritional Values: (per serving)

- Calories: 150
- Protein: 5g
- Fat: 7g

- Carbohydrates: 20g
- Fiber: 6g

Cooking Time: 20 minutes

Serves: 4

Rating: ★★★★★

Tuna Salad Stuffed Avocados

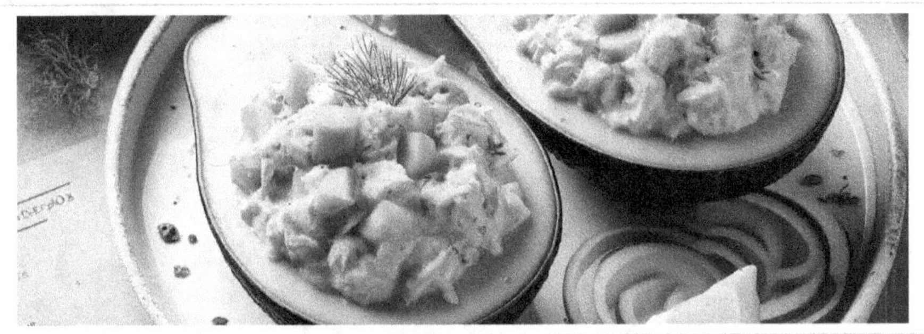

Ingredients:

- 2 avocados, halved and pitted
- 1 can (5 oz) tuna, drained
- 2 tablespoons mayonnaise
- 1/4 cup celery, chopped

- 2 tablespoons red onion, diced
- Juice of 1/2 lemon
- Fresh dill for garnish
- Salt and pepper to taste
- Lettuce leaves for serving

Preparation:

1. In a bowl, mix tuna, mayonnaise, celery, red onion, and lemon juice. Season with salt and pepper.
2. Scoop out a small portion of each avocado half to create space for the tuna salad.
3. Fill each avocado half with the tuna mixture.
4. Garnish with fresh dill.
5. Serve on lettuce leaves.

Nutritional Values: (per serving)

- Calories: 320
- Protein: 15g
- Fat: 25g
- Carbohydrates: 12g
- Fiber: 7g

Cooking Time: 10 minutes

Serves: 4

Rating: ★★★★★

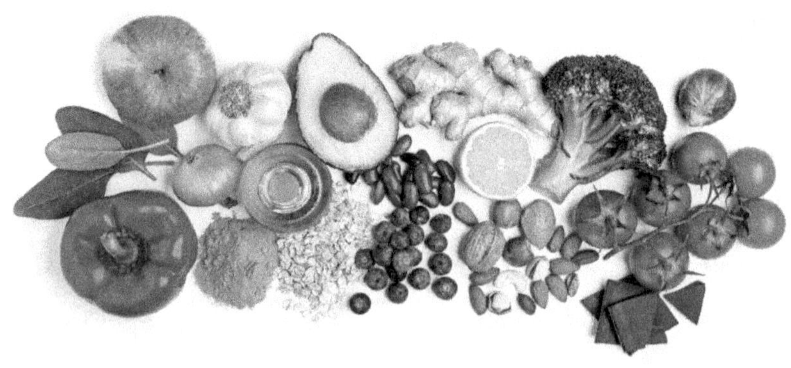

Dinner

Our evening menu is a celebration of tastes that please the tongue while keeping your health in mind. As the sun sets, these meals give comforting warmth and nutritious balance, which are vital for finishing the day on a high note. Each recipe is designed to help persons with insulin resistance, with a focus on healthy ingredients and blood sugar-friendly options. From exquisite grilled salmon to robust vegetable stews, our dinners are intended to be both fun and nourishing, allowing you to unwind and replenish with each bite.

Grilled Salmon with Asparagus

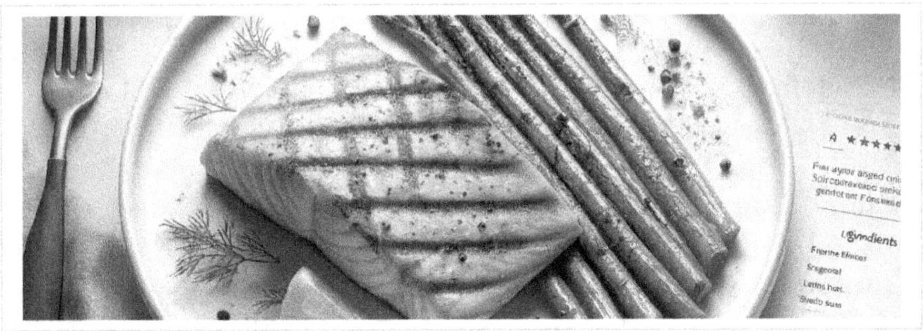

Ingredients:

- 2 salmon fillets
- 1 bunch asparagus, trimmed

- 2 tablespoons olive oil
- 1 lemon, cut into wedges
- Fresh dill, for garnish
- Salt and pepper, to taste

Preparation:

1. Preheat the grill to medium-high heat.
2. Brush the salmon and asparagus with olive oil. Season with salt and pepper.
3. Grill the salmon for about 4 minutes per side or until desired doneness.
4. Grill the asparagus alongside the salmon until tender, about 5 minutes.
5. Serve the salmon and asparagus with lemon wedges and garnish with dill.

Nutritional Values: (per serving)

- Calories: 300
- Protein: 23g
- Fat: 20g
- Carbohydrates: 5g
- Fiber: 2g

Cooking Time: 20 minutes

Serves: 2

Rating: ★★★★★

Chicken Stir-Fry with Broccoli

Ingredients:

- 2 chicken breasts, thinly sliced
- 2 cups broccoli florets
- 1 red bell pepper, sliced
- 1 onion, sliced
- 2 cloves garlic, minced
- 1 inch ginger, minced
- 2 tablespoons soy sauce
- 1 tablespoon olive oil
- Sesame seeds for garnish
- Sliced green onions for garnish

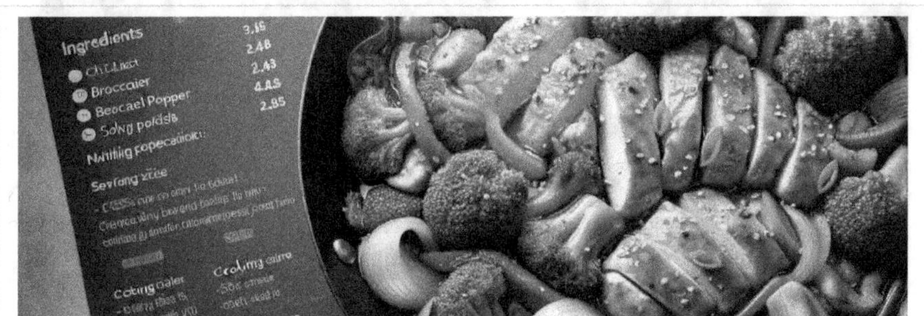

Preparation:

1. Heat olive oil in a wok or large skillet over medium-high heat.
2. Add chicken slices and stir-fry until lightly browned.
3. Add garlic, ginger, broccoli, bell pepper, and onion. Stir-fry for about 5 minutes.
4. Pour soy sauce over the mixture and stir well to coat.
5. Cook for another 2-3 minutes until vegetables are tender but still crisp.
6. Garnish with sesame seeds and green onions.

Nutritional Values: (per serving)

- Calories: 220
- Protein: 26g

- Fat: 7g
- Carbohydrates: 15g

- Fiber: 3g

Cooking Time: 20 minutes

Serves: 4

Rating: ★★★★★

Beef and Vegetable Skewers

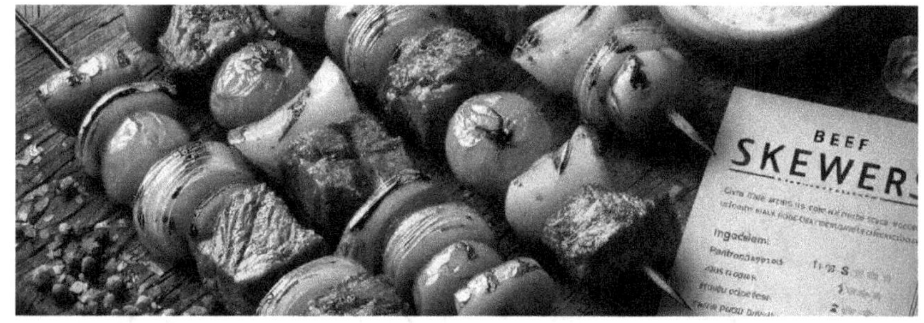

Ingredients:

- 1 lb beef cubes
- 1 red bell pepper, cut into chunks
- 1 green bell pepper, cut into chunks

- 1 zucchini, sliced
- 1 onion, cut into chunks
- 2 tablespoons olive oil
- Salt and pepper to taste

Preparation:

1. Preheat grill to medium-high heat.
2. Thread beef, bell peppers, zucchini, and onion onto skewers.
3. Brush skewers with olive oil and season with salt and pepper.
4. Grill skewers, turning occasionally, until beef is cooked to desired doneness, about 10-15 minutes.

Nutritional Values: (per serving)

- Calories: 250
- Carbohydrates: 5g
- Protein: 25g
- Fiber: 1g
- Fat: 15g

Cooking Time: 20 minutes

Serves: 4

Rating: ★★★★★

Eggplant Lasagna

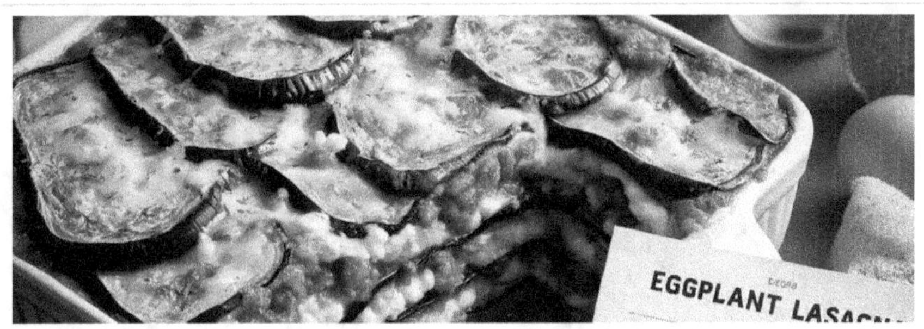

Ingredients:

- 2 large eggplants, sliced lengthwise
- 2 cups shredded mozzarella cheese
- 1 lb ground beef
- 2 tablespoons olive oil
- 2 cups marinara sauce
- 2 cloves garlic, minced
- 1 cup ricotta cheese
- Salt and pepper to taste

Preparation:

1. Preheat oven to 375°F (190°C).

2. Salt eggplant slices and let them sit for 20 minutes to draw out moisture. Rinse and pat dry.

3. Brown ground beef in a skillet with garlic, salt, and pepper.

4. Layer a baking dish with olive oil, then build the lasagna with layers of eggplant, beef mixture, ricotta, marinara sauce, and mozzarella.

5. Bake for 45 minutes, until the top is golden and bubbly.

Nutritional Values: (per serving)

- Calories: 400
- Protein: 25g
- Fat: 25g
- Carbohydrates: 20g
- Fiber: 5g

Cooking Time: 1 hour 10 minutes

Serves: 6

Rating: ★★★★★

Cauliflower Fried Rice

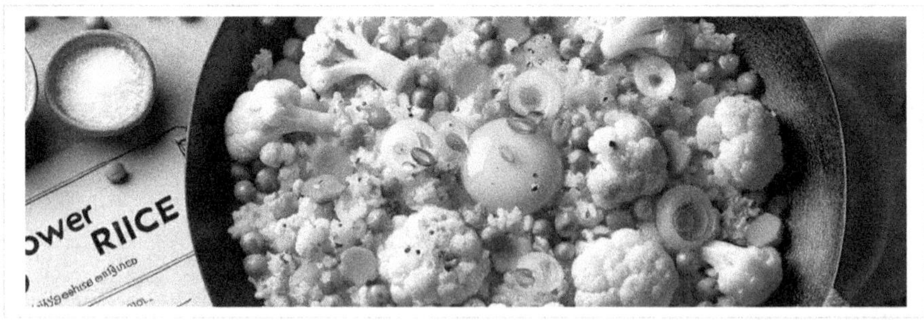

Ingredients:

- 1 head cauliflower, grated
- 1/2 cup peas

- 1/2 cup carrots, diced
- 1 onion, diced
- 2 eggs, beaten
- 2 tablespoons soy sauce
- 1 tablespoon sesame oil
- Salt and pepper to taste
- Green onions and sesame seeds for garnish

Preparation:

1. Heat sesame oil in a large pan over medium heat.
2. Sauté onion, peas, and carrots until soft.
3. Add grated cauliflower and stir-fry for about 5 minutes.
4. Push the vegetables to one side of the pan, add eggs to the other side, and scramble.
5. Mix everything together, add soy sauce, and season with salt and pepper.
6. Garnish with green onions and sesame seeds.

Nutritional Values: (per serving)

- Calories: 180
- Protein: 8g
- Fat: 10g
- Carbohydrates: 15g
- Fiber: 4g

Cooking Time: 20 minutes

Serves: 4

Rating: ★★★★★

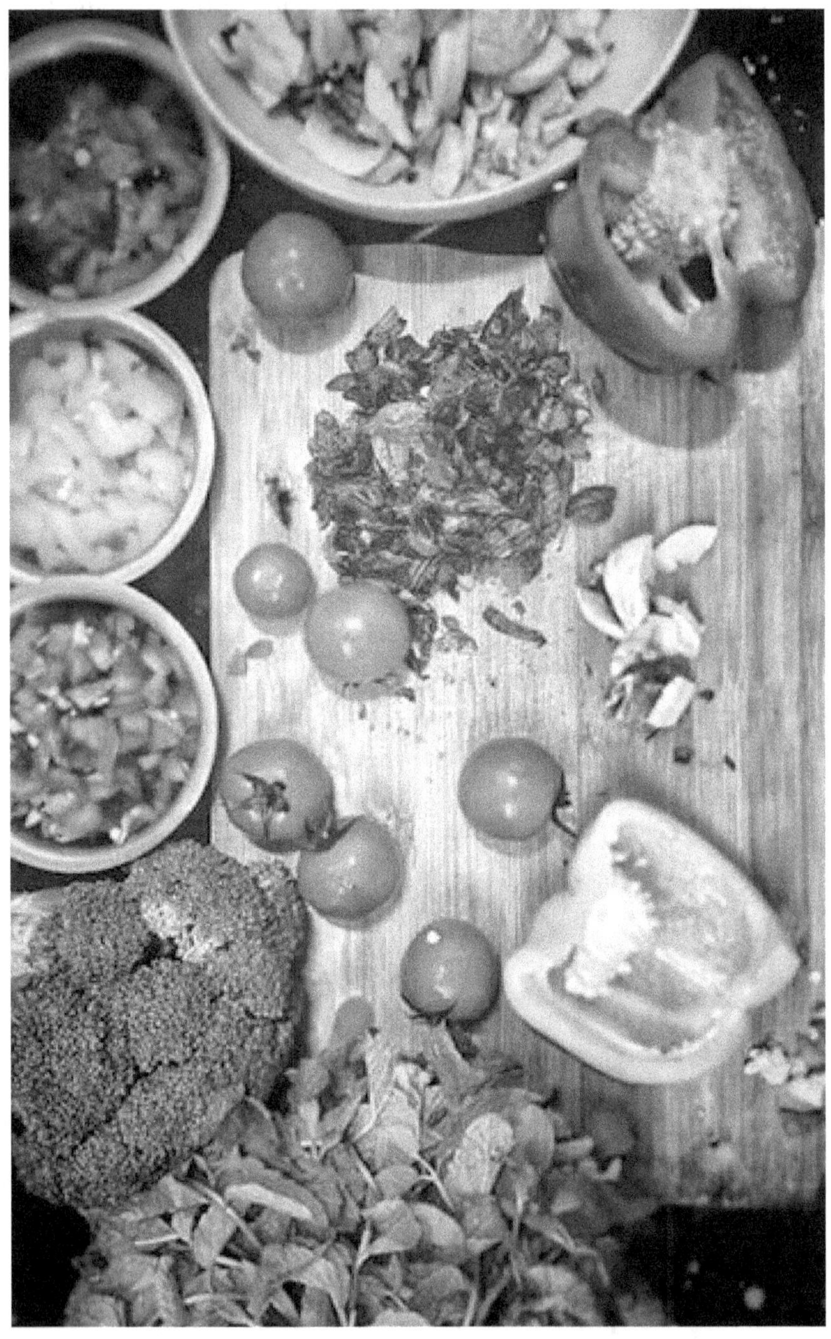

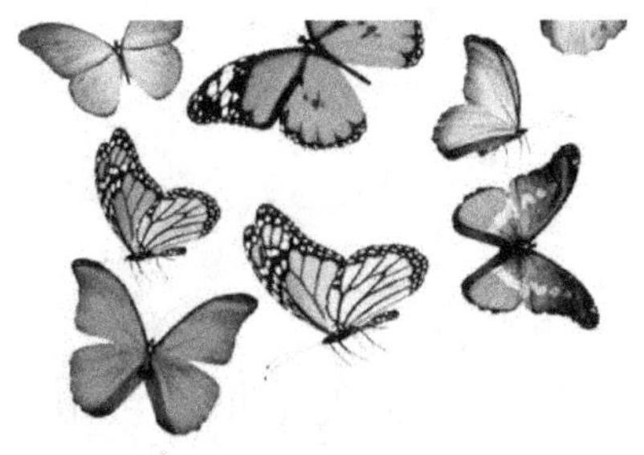

Part 3: Meal Types and Themes

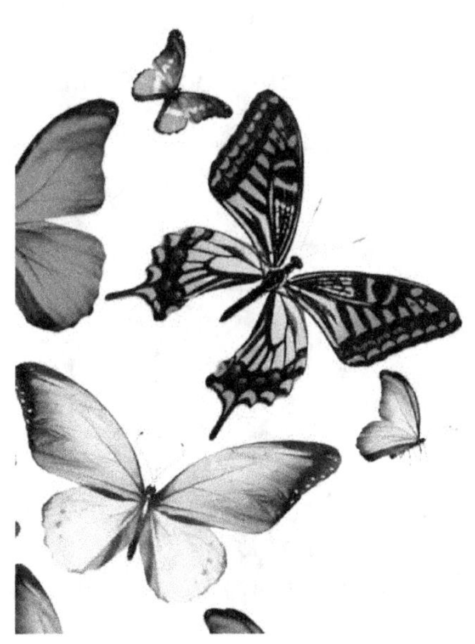

Poultry and Meat

Our cookbook's Poultry and Meat section celebrates the flexibility and nutritional value of lean proteins. Here, we'll look at a variety of delicious, health-conscious meals that will delight your taste buds while also supporting a balanced diet, which is especially useful for individuals dealing with insulin resistance. From luscious chicken dishes and soft turkey compositions to savory beef and lamb recipes, every dish is designed to bring out the most in its components. Whether grilled, roasted, or stir-fried, these protein-packed dishes are enhanced with herbs, spices, and fresh produce to ensure that each bite is not only healthful but also irresistibly delicious. Dive into this section to find dishes that will be the focal point of your dining table, suitable for both ordinary meals and special occasions.

Lemon Herb Chicken

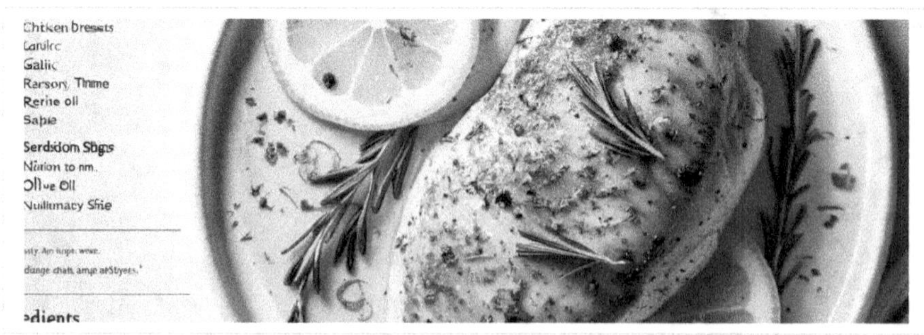

Ingredients:

- 4 chicken breasts
- 2 lemons, one sliced and one juiced
- 4 cloves garlic, minced
- 1 tablespoon rosemary, chopped
- 1 tablespoon thyme, chopped
- 2 tablespoons olive oil
- Salt and pepper to taste

Preparation:

1. Preheat oven to 375°F (190°C).
2. In a bowl, mix lemon juice, olive oil, garlic, rosemary, thyme, salt, and pepper.
3. Place chicken in a baking dish, cover with the marinade, and top with lemon slices.
4. Roast for 25-30 minutes, until chicken is cooked through.
5. Let rest for 5 minutes before serving.

Nutritional Values: (per serving)

- Calories: 220
- Protein: 35g
- Fat: 7g
- Carbohydrates: 3g
- Fiber: 1g

Cooking Time: 35 minutes

Serves: 4

Rating: ★★★★★

Turkey Meatballs in Tomato Sauce

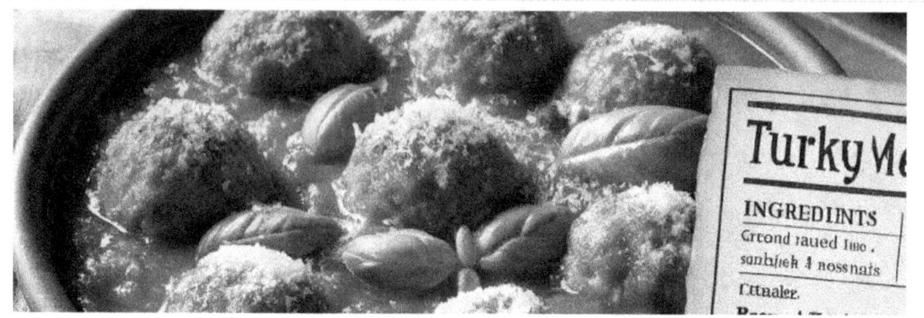

Ingredients:

- 1 lb ground turkey
- 1/2 cup breadcrumbs
- 1 egg
- 2 cloves garlic, minced
- 1 small onion, finely chopped
- 1 can (28 oz) crushed tomatoes
- 1 teaspoon dried basil
- 1 teaspoon dried oregano
- 2 tablespoons grated Parmesan cheese
- 2 tablespoons olive oil
- Salt and pepper to taste
- Fresh basil for garnish

Preparation:

1. Combine ground turkey, breadcrumbs, egg, garlic, half the onion, salt, and pepper in a bowl. Form into meatballs.
2. Heat olive oil in a pan over medium heat. Brown meatballs on all sides and set aside.
3. In the same pan, add the remaining onion and cook until soft. Add crushed tomatoes, basil, and oregano. Bring to a simmer.

4. Return meatballs to the pan, cover, and simmer for 20 minutes.

5. Garnish with Parmesan cheese and fresh basil before serving.

Nutritional Values: (per serving)

- Calories: 320
- Protein: 28g
- Fat: 18g

- Carbohydrates: 12g
- Fiber: 2g

Cooking Time: 40 minutes

Serves: 4

Rating: ★★★★★

Grilled Chicken Caesar Salad

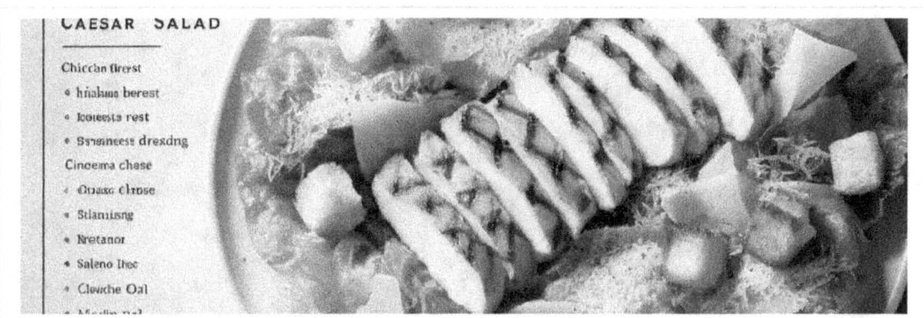

Ingredients:

- 2 chicken breasts, grilled and sliced
- 4 cups romaine lettuce, chopped
- 1 cup croutons

- 1/2 cup shaved Parmesan cheese
- Caesar dressing to taste
- 1 lemon, cut into wedges
- Olive oil for grilling
- Salt and pepper to taste

Preparation:

1. Preheat grill. Brush chicken breasts with olive oil, season with salt and pepper, and grill until cooked through. Slice thinly.
2. Toss romaine lettuce with Caesar dressing in a large bowl.
3. Top the dressed lettuce with grilled chicken slices, croutons, and shaved Parmesan cheese.
4. Serve with lemon wedges on the side.

Nutritional Values: (per serving)

- Calories: 350
- Protein: 30g
- Fat: 20g

- Carbohydrates: 12g
- Fiber: 2g

Cooking Time: 20 minutes

Serves: 4

Rating: ★★★★★

Beef Stroganoff with Zucchini Noodles

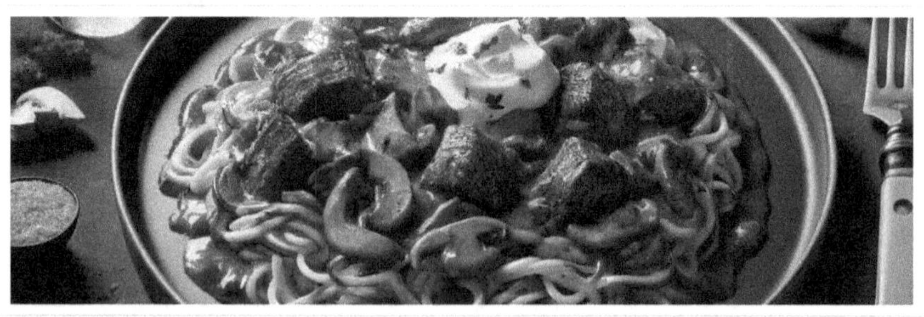

Ingredients:

- 1 lb beef sirloin, thinly sliced
- 2 medium zucchinis, spiralized
- 1 cup mushrooms, sliced
- 1 onion, finely chopped
- 2 cloves garlic, minced
- 1 cup beef broth
- 1/2 cup sour cream
- 1 tablespoon Dijon mustard
- 2 tablespoons olive oil
- Salt and pepper to taste
- Chopped parsley for garnish

Preparation:

1. Heat olive oil in a pan over medium-high heat. Add beef and cook until browned. Set aside.
2. In the same pan, add onions and garlic. Cook until softened.
3. Add mushrooms and cook until browned.
4. Return beef to the pan, add beef broth and Dijon mustard. Simmer until the sauce thickens.
5. Stir in sour cream and heat through. Season with salt and pepper.
6. Serve the stroganoff over spiralized zucchini noodles. Garnish with parsley.

Nutritional Values: (per serving)

- Calories: 320
- Protein: 25g
- Fat: 20g
- Carbohydrates: 8g
- Fiber: 2g

Cooking Time: 30 minutes

Serves: 4   **Rating: ★★★★★**

Pork Tenderloin with Roasted Vegetables

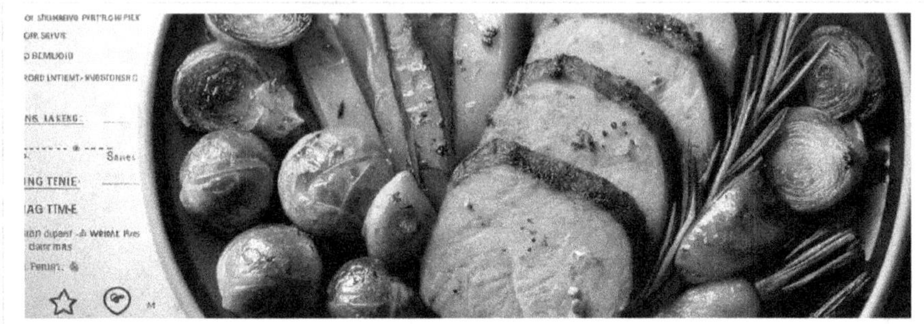

Ingredients:

- 1 pork tenderloin (about 1 lb)
- 2 carrots, peeled and chopped
- 1 cup Brussels sprouts, halved
- 1 sweet potato, peeled and cubed
- 2 tablespoons olive oil
- 2 sprigs rosemary
- Salt and pepper to taste

Preparation:

1. Preheat oven to 425°F (220°C).
2. Season the pork tenderloin with salt and pepper. Place in a roasting pan.
3. Toss the vegetables with olive oil, salt, and pepper. Arrange around the pork.
4. Place rosemary sprigs on top of the pork.

5. Roast for 25-30 minutes, or until the pork reaches an internal temperature of 145°F (63°C).

6. Let the pork rest for 5 minutes before slicing. Serve with the roasted vegetables.

Nutritional Values: (per serving)

- Calories: 310
- Protein: 24g
- Fat: 14g

- Carbohydrates: 22g
- Fiber: 5g

Cooking Time: 35 minutes

Serves: 4

Rating: ★★★★★

Chicken Alfredo with Spaghetti Squash

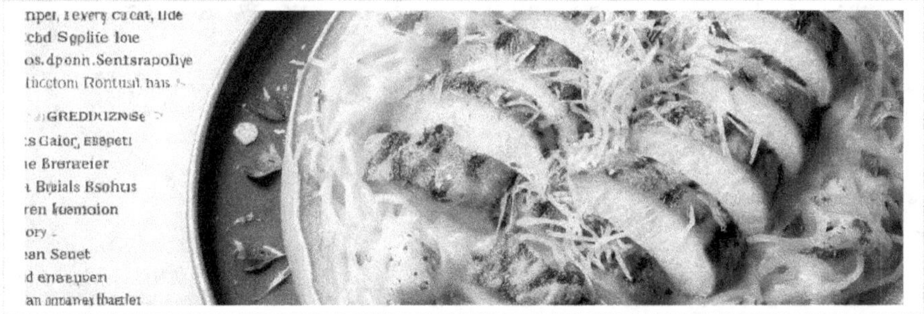

Ingredients:

- 1 large spaghetti squash
- 2 chicken breasts, grilled and sliced
- 1 cup heavy cream

- 1/2 cup grated Parmesan cheese
- 2 tablespoons butter
- 2 cloves garlic, minced

- Salt and pepper to taste
- Parsley for garnish

Preparation:

1. Preheat oven to 400°F (200°C). Halve spaghetti squash and remove seeds. Place cut-side down on a baking sheet and roast until tender, about 40 minutes.
2. Use a fork to scrape the squash strands into "spaghetti."
3. In a saucepan, melt butter over medium heat. Add garlic and sauté until fragrant.
4. Stir in heavy cream and bring to a simmer. Reduce heat and add Parmesan cheese, stirring until the sauce thickens.
5. Season the Alfredo sauce with salt and pepper.
6. Toss spaghetti squash in the Alfredo sauce, top with grilled chicken slices, and garnish with parsley and extra Parmesan.

Nutritional Values: (per serving)

- Calories: 450
- Protein: 30g
- Fat: 32g
- Carbohydrates: 18g
- Fiber: 4g

Cooking Time: 1 hour

Serves: 4

Rating: ★★★★★

Meatloaf with Hidden Veggies

Ingredients:

- 1 lb ground beef
- 1/2 cup breadcrumbs
- 2 eggs
- 1 carrot, finely grated
- 1 zucchini, finely grated
- 1 bell pepper, finely diced
- 1 onion, finely chopped
- 2 cloves garlic, minced
- 1/2 cup tomato sauce (for topping)
- 1 tablespoon Worcestershire sauce
- Salt and pepper to taste

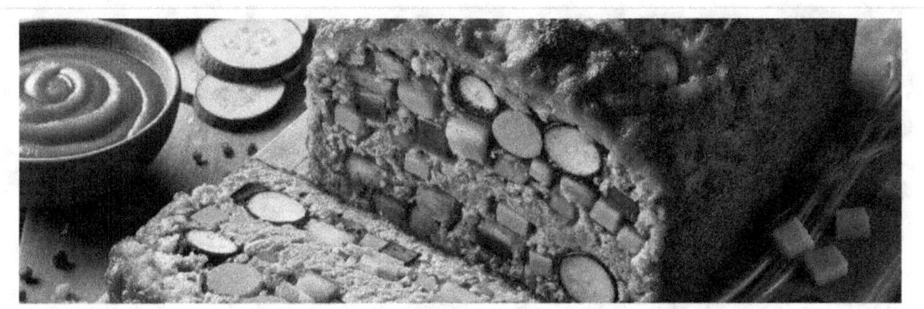

Preparation:

1. Preheat oven to 375°F (190°C).
2. In a large bowl, combine ground beef, breadcrumbs, eggs, grated carrot, zucchini, bell pepper, onion, garlic, Worcestershire sauce, salt, and pepper.
3. Mix well and shape into a loaf on a baking sheet.
4. Top with tomato sauce.
5. Bake for 1 hour or until cooked through.
6. Let rest for 10 minutes before slicing.

Nutritional Values: (per serving)

- Calories: 260
- Protein: 20g
- Fat: 15g
- Carbohydrates: 12g
- Fiber: 2g

Cooking Time: 1 hour 10 minutes

Serves: 6

Rating: ★★★★★

Lamb Chops with Mint Pesto

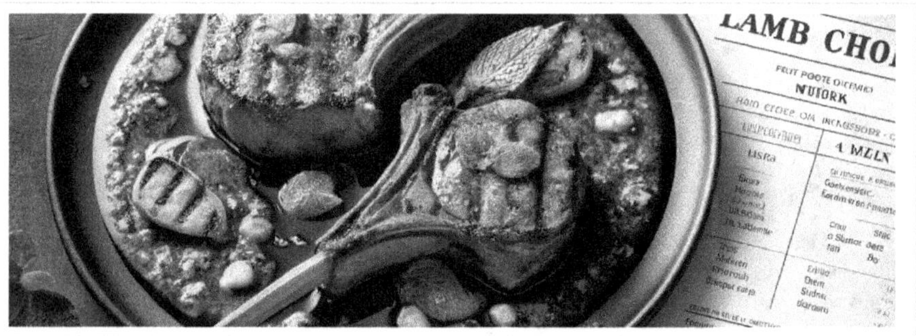

Ingredients:

- 4 lamb chops
- 1 cup fresh mint leaves
- 2 cloves garlic
- 1/4 cup grated Parmesan cheese
- 1/4 cup pine nuts
- 1/3 cup olive oil
- 1 tablespoon lemon juice
- Salt and pepper to taste

Preparation:

1. Season lamb chops with salt and pepper. Grill over medium-high heat to desired doneness.

2. For the mint pesto, blend mint leaves, garlic, Parmesan, pine nuts, lemon juice, and olive oil in a food processor until smooth.

3. Drizzle mint pesto over grilled lamb chops before serving.

Nutritional Values: (per serving)

- Calories: 450
- Protein: 24g
- Fat: 38g

- Carbohydrates: 3g
- Fiber: 1g

Cooking Time: 20 minutes

Serves: 4

Rating: ★★★★★

Baked Chicken Parmesan

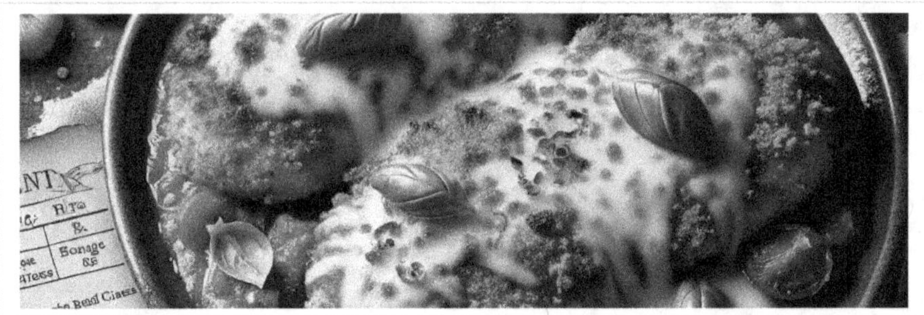

Ingredients:

- 4 chicken breasts
- 1 cup breadcrumbs
- 1/2 cup grated Parmesan cheese
- 1 cup tomato sauce

- 1 cup shredded mozzarella cheese
- 2 eggs, beaten
- 1/2 cup all-purpose flour
- 2 tablespoons olive oil

- Salt and pepper to taste
- Fresh basil for garnish

Preparation:

1. Preheat oven to 400°F (200°C).
2. Season chicken with salt and pepper, dredge in flour, dip in beaten eggs, then coat with a mixture of breadcrumbs and Parmesan.
3. Place chicken on a greased baking sheet, drizzle with olive oil, and bake for 20 minutes.
4. Top each breast with tomato sauce and mozzarella, bake until cheese is melted, about 10 minutes.
5. Garnish with fresh basil before serving.

Nutritional Values: (per serving)

- Calories: 490
- Carbohydrates: 30g
- Protein: 40g
- Fiber: 2g
- Fat: 22g

Cooking Time: 30 minutes

Serves: 4

Rating: ★★★★★

Slow-Cooked Pulled Pork

Ingredients:

- 4 lb pork shoulder
- 2 tablespoons paprika
- 1/4 cup brown sugar

- 1 tablespoon garlic powder
- 1 tablespoon onion powder
- 1 teaspoon salt
- 1 teaspoon pepper
- 1/2 cup apple cider vinegar
- 1 cup barbecue sauce

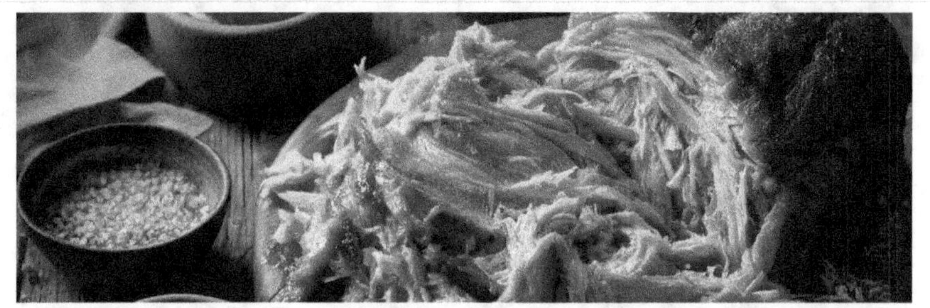

Preparation:

1. Mix brown sugar, paprika, garlic powder, onion powder, salt, and pepper. Rub this mixture all over the pork shoulder.
2. Place the pork in a slow cooker. Pour apple cider vinegar around the pork.
3. Cook on low for 8 hours or until the pork is tender and shreds easily.
4. Shred the pork using two forks. Mix in barbecue sauce.
5. Serve hot with extra sauce on the side.

Nutritional Values: (per serving)

- Calories: 380
- Protein: 25g
- Fat: 25g
- Carbohydrates: 15g

- Fiber: 1g

Cooking Time: 8 hours

Serves: 8   **Rating:** ★★★★★

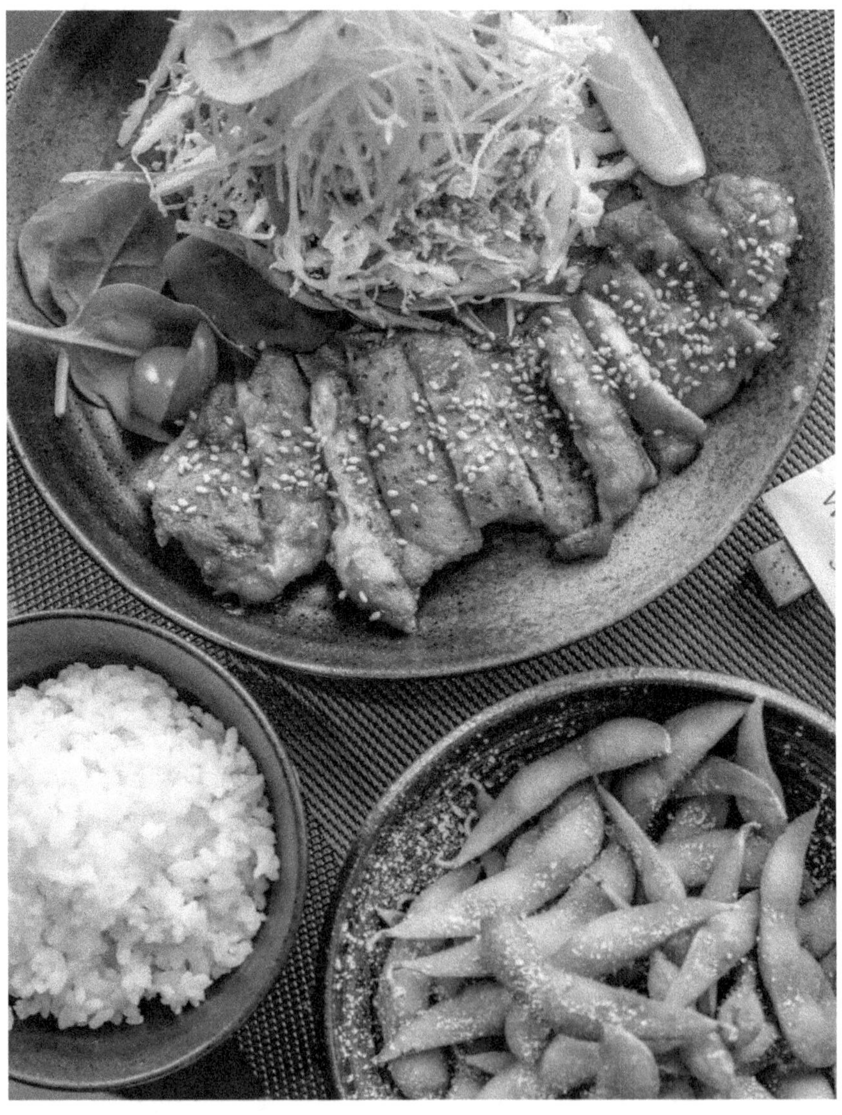

Seafoods and Fish

Explore our cookbook's Seafoods & Fish section, where we highlight the abundance of the sea with a selection of delectable recipes made for those who are concerned about their health, especially those who are managing insulin resistance. This section offers everything from light and zesty salads to rich and soothing stews, all to bring the freshness of the sea directly to your table. We highlight the nutritional advantages of seafood, which is high in proteins, important nutrients, and omega-3 fatty acids, by using a range of cooking methods that maintain the distinct tastes and textures of each fish and shellfish. These dishes, which offer a delectable way to savor the beneficial treasures of the ocean, are designed to satisfy your senses and feed your body, whether you're a fan of salmon, cod, shrimp, or clams.

Shrimp Scampi with Zoodles

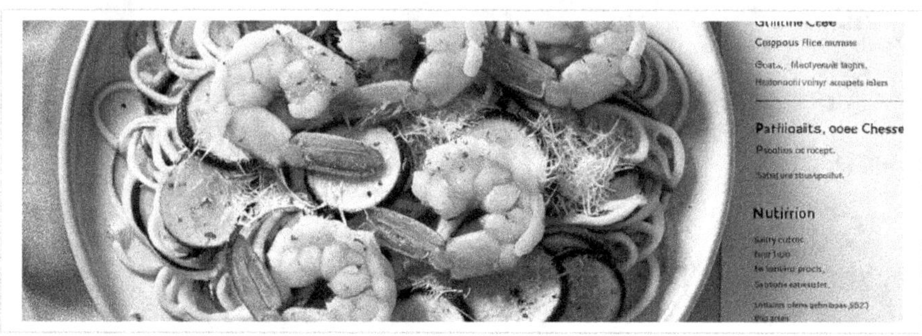

Ingredients:

- 1 lb shrimp, peeled and deveined
- 4 zucchinis, spiralized into noodles
- 4 cloves garlic, minced
- 4 tablespoons butter
- Juice of 1 lemon
- 1/4 cup grated Parmesan cheese
- 2 tablespoons olive oil
- Salt and pepper to taste
- Fresh parsley, chopped for garnish

Preparation:

1. Heat olive oil in a large pan over medium heat. Add garlic and sauté until fragrant.
2. Add shrimp, season with salt and pepper, and cook until pink and opaque.
3. Stir in butter and lemon juice, cook for an additional minute.
4. Toss with zucchini noodles until well combined and heated through.
5. Serve topped with grated Parmesan and fresh parsley.

Nutritional Values: (per serving)

- Calories: 320
- Protein: 25g
- Fat: 20g
- Carbohydrates: 8g
- Fiber: 2g

Cooking Time: 20 minutes

Serves: 4   **Rating:** ★★★★★

Pan-Seared Scallops with Quinoa

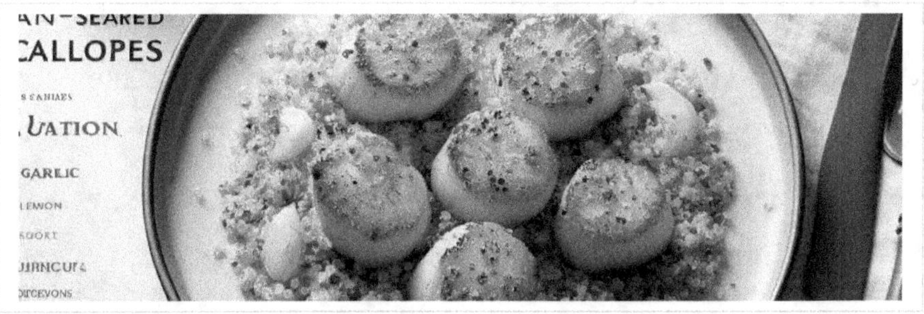

Ingredients:

- 1 lb scallops
- 1 cup quinoa
- 2 cloves garlic, minced
- Juice of 1 lemon
- 2 tablespoons butter
- 1 tablespoon olive oil
- Salt and pepper to taste
- Fresh parsley, chopped for garnish

Preparation:

1. Rinse quinoa under cold water and cook according to package instructions with minced garlic.

2. Heat olive oil in a pan over medium-high heat. Season scallops with salt and pepper, then sear until golden brown on each side, about 1-2 minutes per side.

3. Remove scallops from the pan, add butter and lemon juice to the same pan to make the sauce.

4. Serve scallops over quinoa, drizzle with lemon butter sauce, and garnish with chopped parsley.

Nutritional Values: (per serving)

- Calories: 310
- Protein: 24g
- Fat: 12g

- Carbohydrates: 28g
- Fiber: 3g

Cooking Time: 30 minutes

Serves: 4

Rating: ★★★★★

Baked Cod with Lemon and Dill

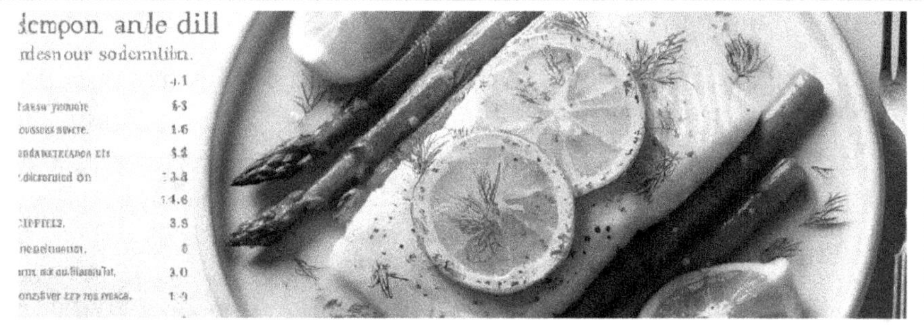

Ingredients:

- 4 cod fillets
- 2 lemons, one sliced and one juiced
- 2 tablespoons fresh dill, chopped

- 2 tablespoons olive oil
- Salt and pepper to taste
- Asparagus for garnish

Preparation:

1. Preheat oven to 400°F (200°C).

2. Place cod fillets in a baking dish. Drizzle with olive oil and lemon juice. Season with salt and pepper.

3. Arrange lemon slices on top of the cod and sprinkle with dill.

4. Bake for 12-15 minutes, until cod is flaky and opaque.

5. Serve with steamed asparagus on the side.

Nutritional Values: (per serving)

- Calories: 200
- Protein: 23g
- Fat: 10g
- Carbohydrates: 3g
- Fiber: 1g

Cooking Time: 15 minutes

Serves: 4

Rating: ★★★★★

Salmon Burgers

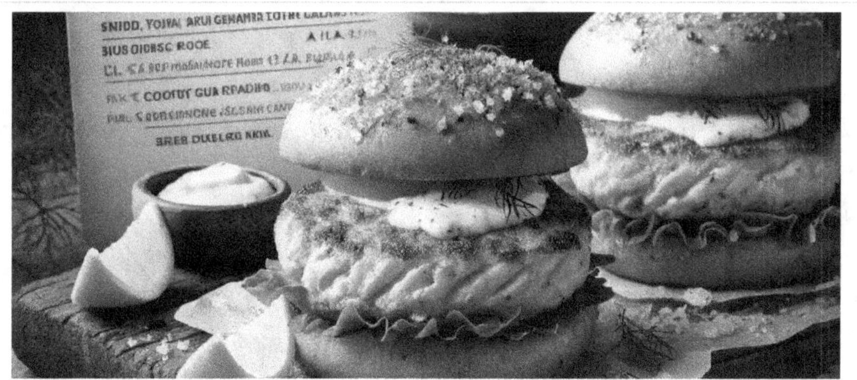

Ingredients:

- 1 lb salmon fillets, finely chopped
- 1/2 cup breadcrumbs
- 1 egg
- 1 lemon, zest and juice
- 2 tablespoons fresh dill, chopped
- 1/2 cup Greek yogurt
- 4 whole-grain buns
- 2 sweet potatoes, cut into fries
- Mixed greens for salad
- Olive oil for cooking
- Salt and pepper to taste

Preparation:

1. Mix salmon, breadcrumbs, egg, lemon zest, salt, and pepper. Form into patties.
2. Grill patties over medium heat until cooked through, about 4 minutes per side.
3. Mix yogurt with lemon juice and dill for the sauce.
4. Toss sweet potato fries with olive oil, salt, and pepper. Bake at 425°F (220°C) until crispy.
5. Assemble burgers with salmon patties, dill yogurt sauce, and buns. Serve with sweet potato fries and salad.

Nutritional Values: (per serving)

- Calories: 450
- Protein: 30g
- Fat: 20g
- Carbohydrates: 40g
- Fiber: 5g

Cooking Time: 30 minutes

Serves: 4   **Rating:** ★★★★★

Tuna Nicoise Salad

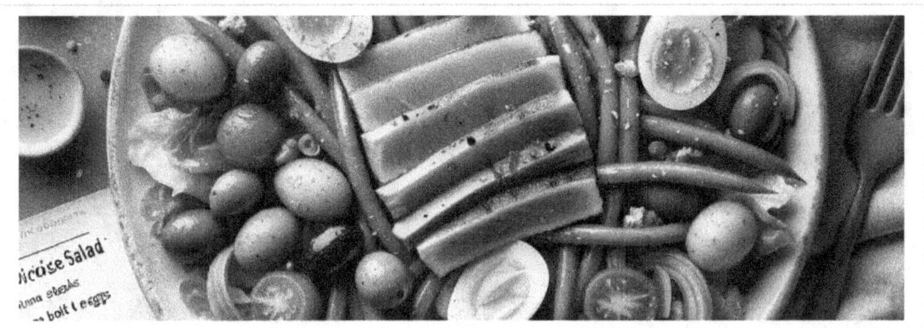

Ingredients:

- 2 tuna steaks
- 1 cup green beans, trimmed
- 4 hard-boiled eggs, quartered
- 1 cup cherry tomatoes, halved
- 1/2 cup black olives
- 1 cup new potatoes, boiled and halved
- 4 cups mixed greens
- For the dressing:
  - 3 tablespoons olive oil
  - 1 tablespoon vinegar
  - 1 teaspoon mustard
  - Salt and pepper to taste

Preparation:

1. Season tuna steaks with salt and pepper. Sear over high heat to desired doneness. Slice thinly.

2. Blanch green beans in boiling water for 2 minutes. Refresh in ice water.

3. Arrange mixed greens on a plate. Top with tuna, green beans, eggs, tomatoes, olives, and potatoes.

4. Whisk together dressing ingredients and drizzle over the salad.

Nutritional Values: (per serving)

- Calories: 400
- Protein: 35g
- Fat: 20g
- Carbohydrates: 20g
- Fiber: 5g

Cooking Time: 30 minutes

Serves: 4

Rating: ★★★★★

Grilled Mackerel with Salsa Verde

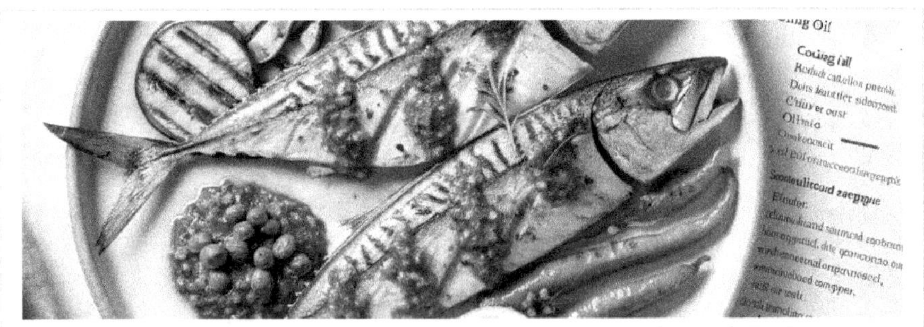

Ingredients:

- 4 mackerel fillets
- For the salsa verde:
- 1/2 cup parsley, chopped

- 1/4 cup basil, chopped
- 1/4 cup mint, chopped
- 2 tablespoons capers, chopped
- 1 clove garlic, minced
- Juice of 1 lemon
- 1/3 cup olive oil
- Assorted grilled vegetables (zucchini, bell peppers, cherry tomatoes)
- Salt and pepper to taste

Preparation:

1. Preheat the grill to medium-high heat.
2. Season mackerel fillets with salt and pepper. Grill until cooked through, about 3-4 minutes per side.
3. For the salsa verde, mix parsley, basil, mint, capers, garlic, lemon juice, and olive oil in a bowl. Season with salt and pepper.
4. Serve grilled mackerel topped with salsa verde and a side of grilled vegetables.

Nutritional Values: (per serving)

- Calories: 350
- Protein: 25g
- Fat: 26g
- Carbohydrates: 5g
- Fiber: 2g

Cooking Time: 20 minutes

Serves: 4

Rating: ★★★★★

Fish Tacos with Cabbage Slaw

Ingredients:

- 1 lb white fish (cod or tilapia)
- 8 corn tortillas
- 2 cups shredded cabbage
- 1 carrot, julienned
- 1/4 cup mayonnaise
- 1/4 cup sour cream
- 1 lime, juiced
- 1/4 cup cilantro, chopped
- 1/2 cup flour
- 1/2 cup beer
- 2 tablespoons olive oil
- Salt and pepper to taste
- Avocado slices and lime wedges for garnish

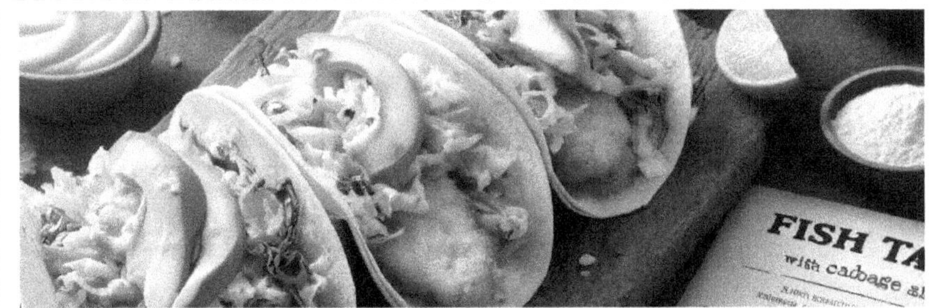

Preparation:

1. Combine flour, beer, salt, and pepper to make a batter. Dip fish in batter and fry in olive oil until golden.
2. Mix cabbage, carrot, mayonnaise, sour cream, lime juice, and cilantro to make the slaw.
3. Warm tortillas in a skillet.
4. Assemble tacos with fish, slaw, and avocado slices. Serve with lime wedges.

Nutritional Values: (per serving)

- Calories: 400
- Protein: 25g
- Fat: 20g

- Carbohydrates: 35g
- Fiber: 5g

Cooking Time: 30 minutes

Serves: 4

Rating: ★★★★★

Crab Cakes with Aioli Sauce

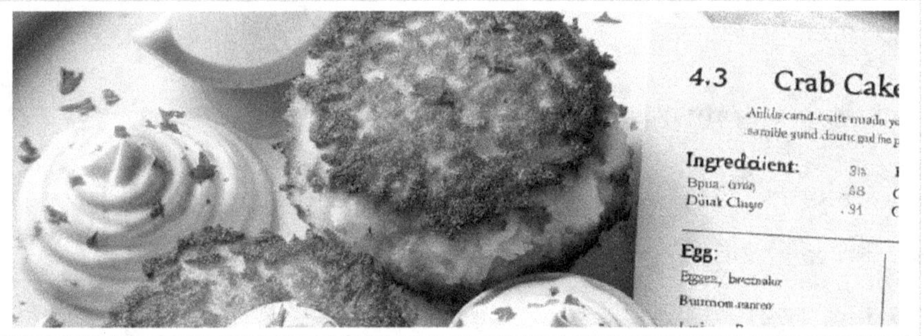

Ingredients:

- 1 lb crab meat
- 1 cup breadcrumbs
- 1/4 cup mayonnaise
- 2 eggs
- 1 tablespoon Dijon mustard
- 2 cloves garlic, minced
- Juice of 1 lemon

- 2 tablespoons olive oil
- Salt and pepper to taste
- For Aioli Sauce:
  - 1/2 cup mayonnaise
  - 1 clove garlic, minced
  - 2 tablespoons lemon juice
  - Salt and pepper to taste

Preparation:

1. Mix crab meat, breadcrumbs, mayonnaise, eggs, mustard, garlic, lemon juice, salt, and pepper. Form into patties.
2. Heat olive oil in a pan and cook crab cakes until golden on each side.
3. For the aioli, combine mayonnaise, garlic, lemon juice, salt, and pepper.
4. Serve crab cakes with aioli sauce and garnish with parsley and lemon wedges.

Nutritional Values: (per serving)

- Calories: 310
- Protein: 24g
- Fat: 18g
- Carbohydrates: 12g
- Fiber: 1g

Cooking Time: 20 minutes

Serves: 4

Rating: ★★★★★

Seafood Paella with Cauliflower Rice

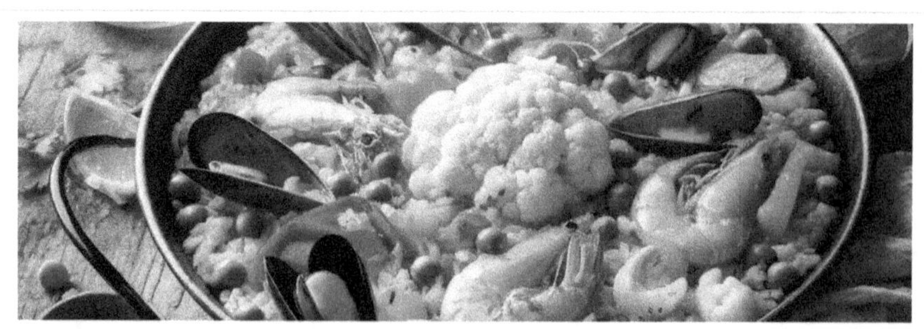

Ingredients:

- 1 head of cauliflower, riced
- 1/2 lb shrimp, peeled and deveined
- 1/2 lb mussels, cleaned
- 1/2 lb clams, cleaned
- 1 red bell pepper, sliced
- 1 green bell pepper, sliced
- 1/2 cup peas
- 1 teaspoon saffron threads
- 1 teaspoon smoked paprika
- 2 tablespoons olive oil
- Salt and pepper to taste
- Lemon wedges and fresh parsley for garnish

Preparation:

1. Heat olive oil in a large pan over medium heat. Add the bell peppers and sauté until soft.
2. Stir in the cauliflower rice, saffron, and smoked paprika. Cook for about 5 minutes.
3. Add the shrimp, mussels, and clams. Cover and cook until the shellfish open and the shrimp are cooked through, about 10 minutes.
4. Stir in the peas and cook for an additional 2 minutes.
5. Season with salt and pepper. Garnish with lemon wedges and fresh parsley before serving.

Nutritional Values: (per serving)

- Calories: 290
- Protein: 25g

- Fat: 12g
- Carbohydrates: 15g

- Fiber: 5g

Cooking Time: 25 minutes

Serves: 4

Rating: ★★★★★

Baked Tilapia with Olives and Tomatoes

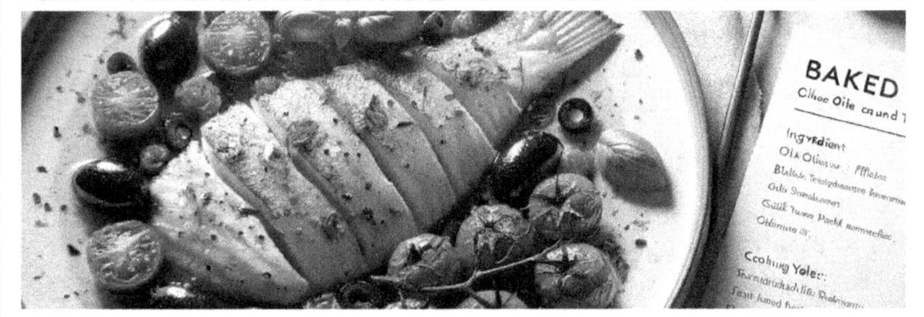

Ingredients:

- 4 tilapia fillets
- 1 cup cherry tomatoes, halved
- 1/2 cup black olives, sliced

- 3 tablespoons olive oil
- 2 cloves garlic, minced
- Fresh basil, for garnish
- Salt and pepper to taste

Preparation:

1. Preheat oven to 400°F (200°C).
2. Arrange tilapia fillets in a baking dish. Season with salt and pepper.
3. Scatter cherry tomatoes and olives around the fish.
4. Drizzle with olive oil and sprinkle with minced garlic.

5. Bake for 15-20 minutes, until fish is flaky.

6. Garnish with fresh basil before serving.

Nutritional Values: (per serving)

- Calories: 220
- Protein: 23g
- Fat: 12g

- Carbohydrates: 5g
- Fiber: 1g

Cooking Time: 20 minutes

Serves: 4

Rating: ★★★★★

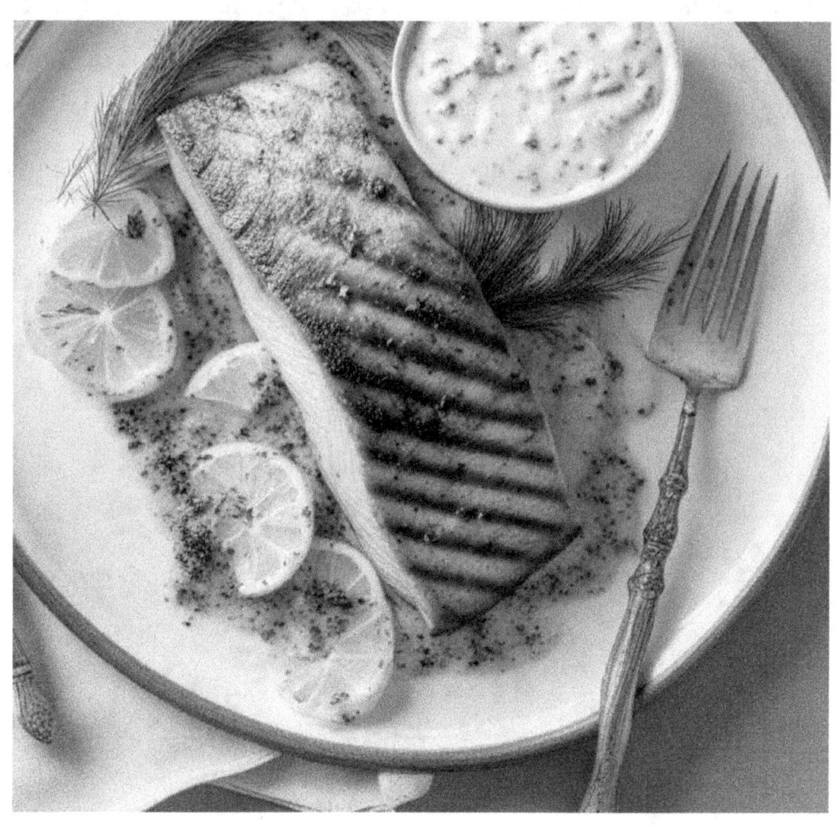

Snacks

This section focuses on snacks that not only fulfill your cravings but also give long-term energy and nutritional benefits—particularly crucial for managing insulin resistance. These recipes are designed to provide delicious, practical, and healthful solutions that can easily be included in your daily routine. Each snack, from savory goodies like handmade kale chips and protein-rich nut mixes to sweet treats like yogurt parfaits and fresh fruit salads, is designed to provide a balance of proteins, healthy fats, and fibers to help regulate blood sugar levels and keep you feeling fuller for longer. Whether you need a fast afternoon pick-me-up or a post-workout boost, these snacks are ideal for maintaining your energy levels without sacrificing taste or health.

Cucumber and Hummus Bites

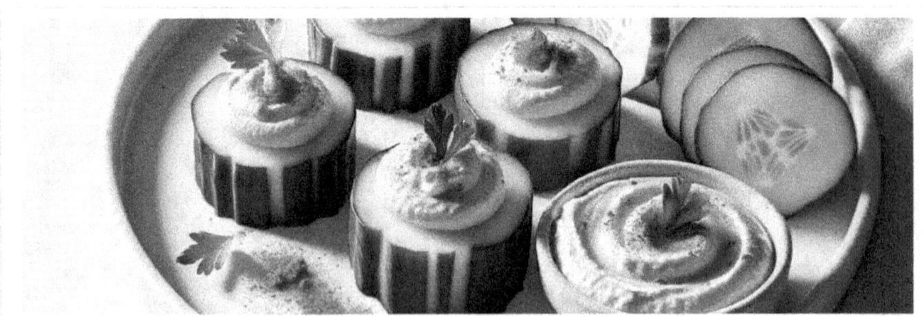

Ingredients:

- 2 large cucumbers, sliced into rounds
- 1 cup hummus
- Paprika for sprinkling
- Fresh parsley leaves for garnish

Preparation:

1. Slice cucumbers into thick rounds.
2. Top each cucumber slice with a spoonful of hummus.
3. Sprinkle a little paprika over the hummus and garnish with a parsley leaf.

Nutritional Values: (per serving)

- Calories: 35
- Protein: 2g
- Fat: 2g
- Carbohydrates: 3g
- Fiber: 1g

Cooking Time: 10 minutes

Serves: 4

Rating: ★★★★☆

Almonds and Cheese

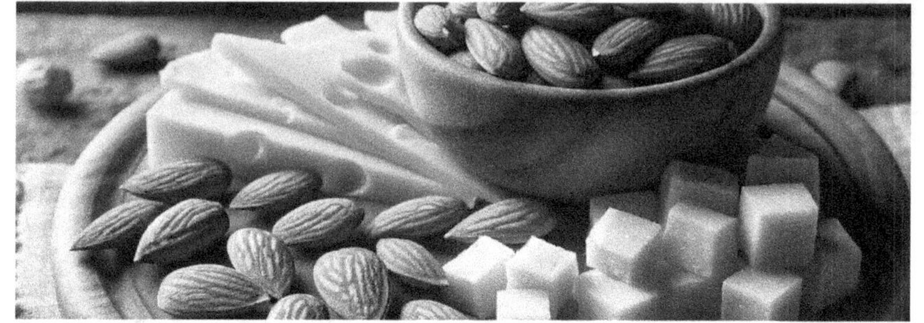

Ingredients:

- 1 cup whole almonds
- 1 cup cheddar cheese, cubed

Preparation:

1. Arrange whole almonds and cubes of cheddar cheese on a serving board.

Nutritional Values: (per serving)

- Calories: 250
- Carbohydrates: 6g
- Protein: 12g
- Fiber: 3g
- Fat: 20g

Cooking Time: None

Serves: 4

Rating: ★★★★☆

Greek Yogurt with Berries

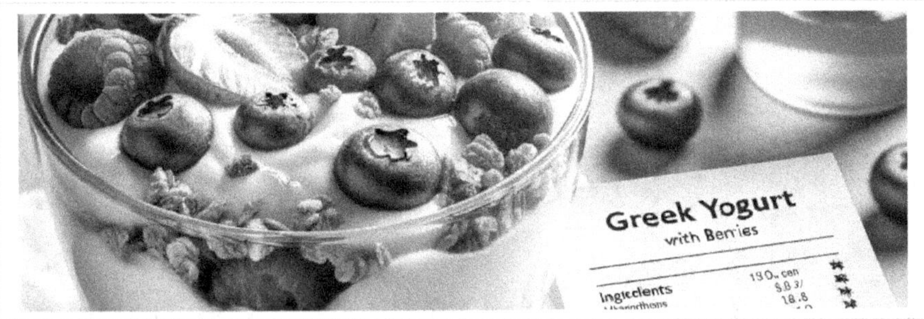

Ingredients:

- 1 cup Greek yogurt
- 1/2 cup mixed berries (blueberries, raspberries, strawberries)

- 1 tablespoon honey
- 1/4 cup granola

Preparation:

1. Spoon Greek yogurt into a serving bowl.
2. Top with mixed berries.
3. Drizzle honey over the berries and sprinkle with granola.

Nutritional Values: (per serving)

- Calories: 220
- Carbohydrates: 30g
- Protein: 15g
- Fiber: 3g
- Fat: 6g

Cooking Time: None

Serves: 1

Rating: ★★★★★

Avocado Chocolate Mousse

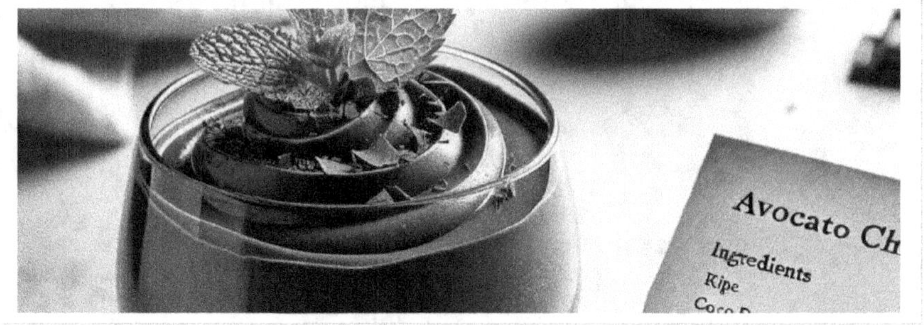

Ingredients:

- 2 ripe avocados
- 1 teaspoon vanilla extract
- 1/4 cup cocoa powder
- Pinch of sea salt
- 1/4 cup maple syrup
- 1/4 cup coconut cream

Preparation:

1. Peel and pit the avocados.
2. Blend avocados, cocoa powder, maple syrup, vanilla extract, and sea salt in a food processor until smooth.
3. Whip the coconut cream separately until light and fluffy.
4. Fold the whipped coconut cream into the avocado mixture gently.
5. Chill in the refrigerator for at least 1 hour before serving.
6. Garnish with a mint leaf and dark chocolate shavings.

Nutritional Values: (per serving)

- Calories: 250
- Protein: 3g
- Fat: 20g
- Carbohydrates: 20g
- Fiber: 7g

Cooking Time: 1 hour 10 minutes (including chilling)

Serves: 4

Rating: ★★★★★

Kale Chips

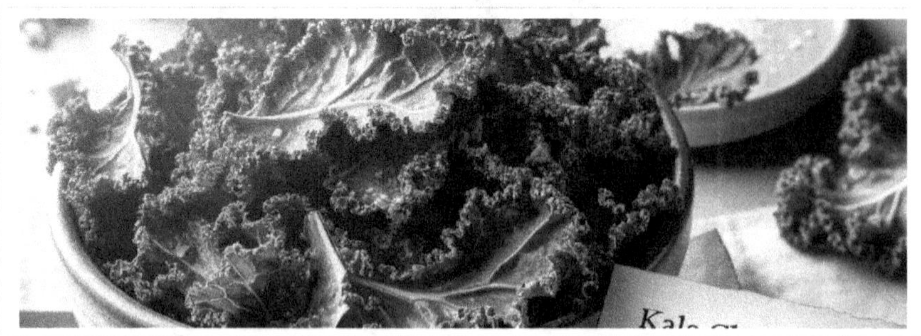

Ingredients:

- 1 bunch kale, washed and torn into bite-size pieces
- 2 tablespoons olive oil
- 1/2 teaspoon sea salt
- 2 tablespoons nutritional yeast

Preparation:

1. Preheat oven to 300°F (150°C).
2. Dry kale thoroughly after washing. In a large bowl, toss kale with olive oil, salt, and nutritional yeast until evenly coated.
3. Spread kale in a single layer on a baking sheet.
4. Bake for about 20 minutes or until crisp, turning halfway through.
5. Let cool before serving to enhance crispiness.

Nutritional Values: (per serving)

- Calories: 150
- Protein: 5g
- Fat: 10g
- Carbohydrates: 10g
- Fiber: 2g

Cooking Time: 20 minutes

Serves: 4

Rating: ★★★★★

Sides

Explore our variety of side dishes that will enhance the flavors of any meal while also adding nutritional balance. Whether you want to round out a family supper, add variety to your lunch, or serve something special alongside a holiday feast, this section has something for everyone. Our sides range from vibrant veggies and healthful grains to luscious creams and light salads, all designed to promote a healthy lifestyle while adding a pop of flavor and color to your plate. These recipes are simple but diverse, allowing you to simply discover the right companion to your main dishes, regardless of dietary concerns or preferences. Enjoy exploring these innovative, delicious, and health-conscious options that guarantee to round out any meal.

Roasted Brussels Sprouts

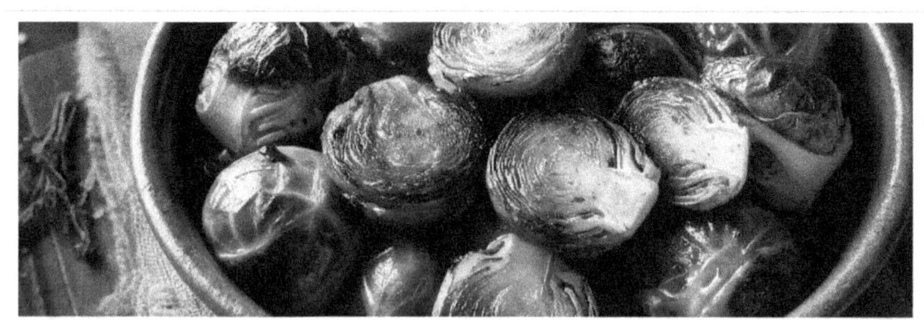

Ingredients:

- lb Brussels sprouts, halved
- 2 tablespoons olive oil
- 1/2 teaspoon sea salt
- 1/4 teaspoon freshly cracked black pepper

Preparation:

1. Preheat oven to 400°F (200°C).
2. Toss Brussels sprouts with olive oil, salt, and pepper.
3. Spread on a baking sheet in a single layer.
4. Roast for 25-30 minutes, stirring halfway through, until crisp and golden.

Nutritional Values: (per serving)

- Calories: 80
- Protein: 3g
- Fat: 5g
- Carbohydrates: 8g
- Fiber: 3g

Cooking Time: 30 minutes

Serves: 4

Rating: ★★★★★

Sweet Potato Fries

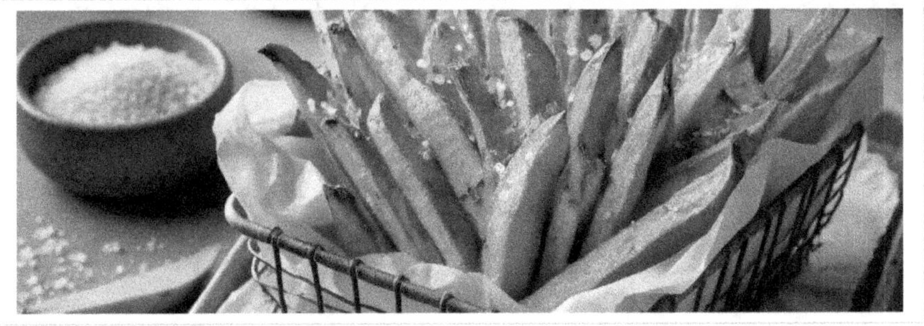

Ingredients:

- 2 large sweet potatoes, peeled and cut into fries
- 2 tablespoons olive oil
- 1/2 teaspoon sea salt
- 1/4 teaspoon smoked paprika

Preparation:

1. Preheat oven to 425°F (220°C).
2. Toss sweet potato fries with olive oil, sea salt, and smoked paprika.
3. Spread on a baking sheet in a single layer.
4. Bake for 25-30 minutes, turning halfway through, until crispy and golden.

Nutritional Values: (per serving)

- Calories: 200
- Protein: 2g
- Fat: 7g
- Carbohydrates: 35g
- Fiber: 5g

Cooking Time: 30 minutes

Serves: 4

Rating: ★★★★★

Garlic Mashed Cauliflower

Ingredients:

- 1 head of cauliflower, cut into florets
- 4 cloves garlic, minced
- 1/4 cup cream

- 2 tablespoons olive oil
- Salt and pepper to taste
- Chives, chopped for garnish

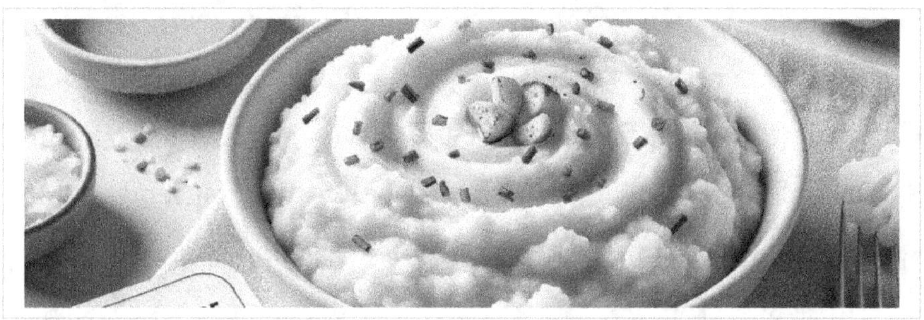

Preparation:

1. Steam cauliflower florets until very tender, about 10 minutes.
2. In a blender or food processor, combine steamed cauliflower, garlic, cream, and olive oil. Puree until smooth.
3. Season with salt and pepper.
4. Serve garnished with chopped chives.

Nutritional Values: (per serving)

- Calories: 150
- Protein: 3g
- Fat: 11g
- Carbohydrates: 10g
- Fiber: 4g

Cooking Time: 20 minutes

Serves: 4

Rating: ★★★★★

Mixed Green Salad with Vinaigrette

Ingredients:

- 2 cups mixed greens (spinach, arugula, romaine)
- 1 cucumber, sliced
- 1 cup cherry tomatoes, halved
- 1/2 red onion, thinly sliced
- 1/4 cup crumbled feta cheese
- 1/4 cup croutons
- For the vinaigrette:
- 3 tablespoons olive oil
- tablespoon balsamic vinegar
- teaspoon mustard
- teaspoon honey
- Salt and pepper to taste

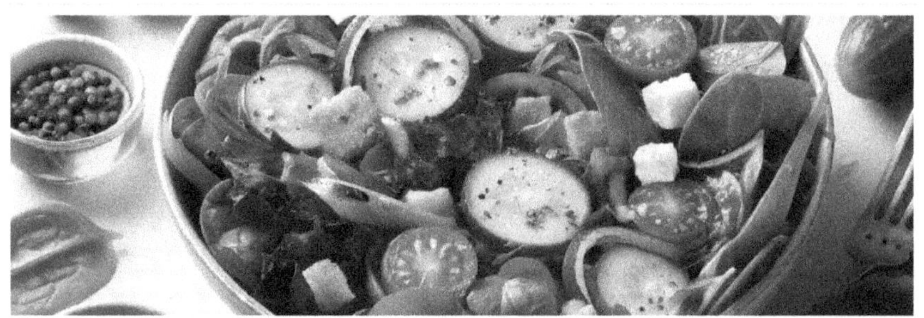

Preparation:

1. In a large bowl, combine mixed greens, cucumber, cherry tomatoes, and red onion.

2. In a small bowl, whisk together olive oil, balsamic vinegar, mustard, honey, salt, and pepper to make the vinaigrette.

3. Drizzle the vinaigrette over the salad and toss to coat evenly.

4. Top with crumbled feta cheese and croutons before serving.

Nutritional Values: (per serving)

- Calories: 180
- Protein: 4g

- Fat: 14g
- Carbohydrates: 12g

- Fiber: 2g

Cooking Time: 10 minutes

Serves: 4

Rating: ★★★★★

Sautéed Green Beans

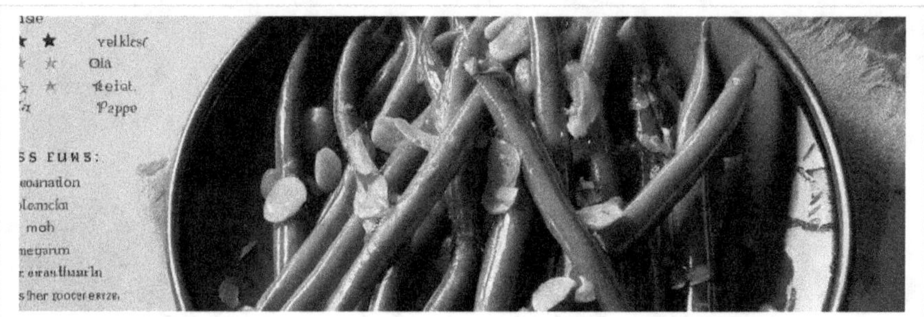

Ingredients:

- 1 lb green beans, trimmed
- 3 cloves garlic, thinly sliced
- 2 tablespoons olive oil

- 1/4 cup slivered almonds, toasted
- Salt and pepper to taste

Preparation:

1. Heat olive oil in a large skillet over medium heat.

2. Add garlic and sauté until fragrant, about 1 minute.

3. Add green beans and cook, stirring occasionally, until tender-crisp, about 5-7 minutes.

4. Season with salt and pepper.

5. Sprinkle with toasted almonds before serving.

Nutritional Values: (per serving)

- Calories: 120
- Protein: 3g
- Fat: 9g

- Carbohydrates: 10g
- Fiber: 4g

Cooking Time: 10 minutes

Serves: 4

Rating: ★★★★★

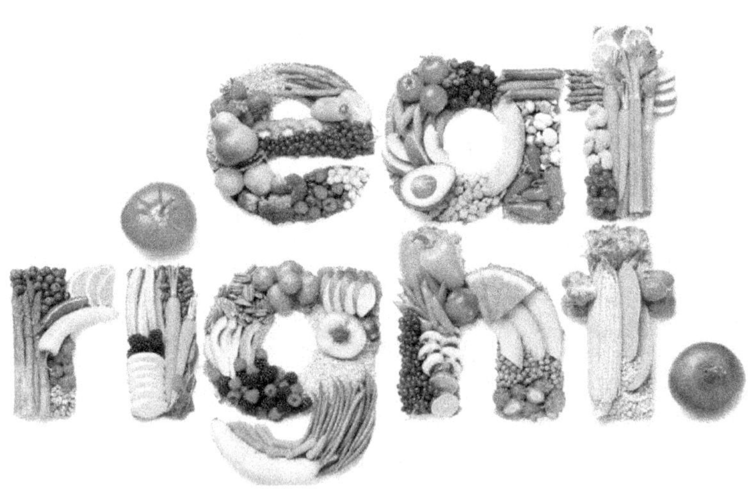

Stews

Explore our stews, which combine rich tastes and soft textures in comforting, one-pot meals. These recipes include meaty classics, savory seafood, and brilliant vegetable stews, all cooked to perfection. These comfortable dishes are ideal for any season, whether you want to warm up on a cold day or fulfill your hunger with nutritious ingredients.

Chicken and Vegetable Stew

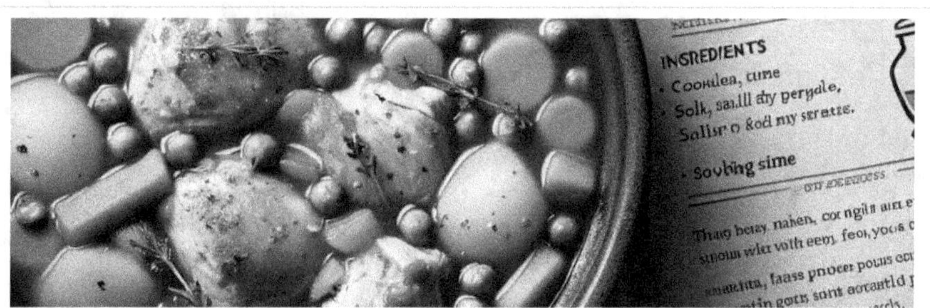

Ingredients:

- 1 lb chicken breasts, cubed
- 2 carrots, peeled and sliced
- 2 potatoes, peeled and cubed
- 1 cup peas
- 4 cups chicken broth
- 1 onion, chopped
- 2 cloves garlic, minced
- 2 tablespoons olive oil

- 1 teaspoon thyme
- Salt and pepper to taste

Preparation:

1. Heat olive oil in a large pot over medium heat.
2. Sauté onions and garlic until translucent.
3. Add chicken and brown slightly.
4. Stir in carrots, potatoes, and thyme, then add chicken broth.
5. Bring to a boil, reduce heat, and simmer for 25 minutes.
6. Add peas and cook for an additional 5 minutes.
7. Season with salt and pepper to taste.

Nutritional Values: (per serving)

- Calories: 300
- Carbohydrates: 30g
- Protein: 28g
- Fiber: 5g
- Fat: 8g

Cooking Time: 40 minutes

Serves: 4

Rating: ★★★★★

Beef Chili

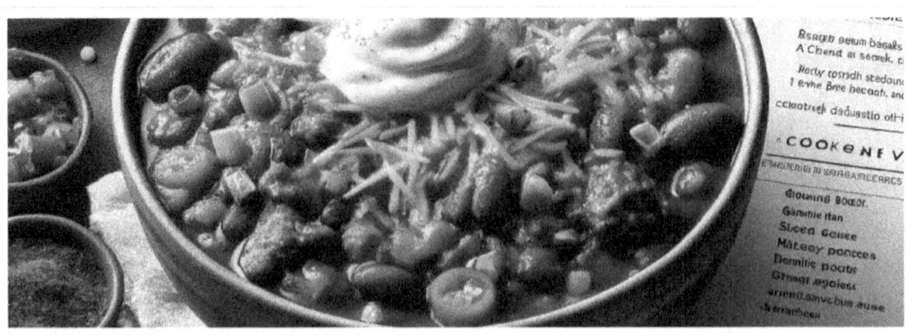

Ingredients:

- 1 lb ground beef
- 1 can kidney beans, drained and rinsed
- 1 can diced tomatoes
- 1 bell pepper, chopped
- 1 onion, chopped
- 2 cloves garlic, minced
- 2 tablespoons chili powder
- 1 teaspoon cumin
- 2 tablespoons olive oil
- Salt and pepper to taste
- Sour cream, shredded cheddar cheese, and chopped green onions for garnish

Preparation:

1. Heat olive oil in a large pot over medium heat.
2. Add onion and garlic, cook until soft.
3. Add ground beef, cook until browned.
4. Stir in bell pepper, kidney beans, diced tomatoes, chili powder, and cumin.
5. Season with salt and pepper, simmer for 30 minutes.
6. Serve topped with sour cream, cheddar cheese, and green onions.

Nutritional Values: (per serving)

- Calories: 400
- Protein: 25g
- Fat: 20g
- Carbohydrates: 30g
- Fiber: 8g

Cooking Time: 40 minutes

Serves: 4   **Rating:** ★★★★★

Lentil Soup

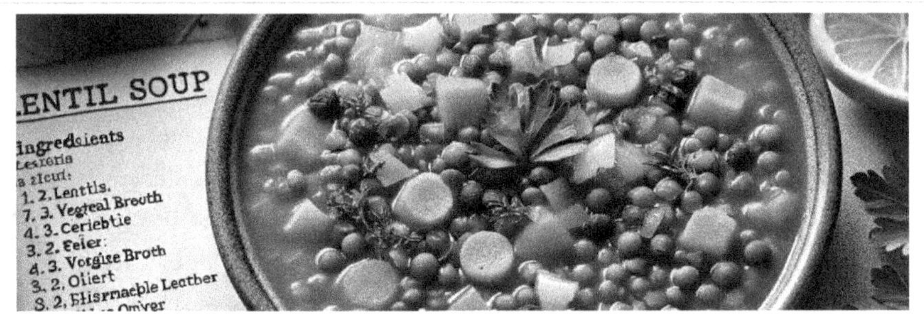

Ingredients:

- 1 cup lentils
- 2 carrots, diced
- 2 celery stalks, diced
- 1 onion, chopped
- 4 cups vegetable broth
- 1 teaspoon dried thyme
- 1 bay leaf
- 2 tablespoons olive oil
- Salt and pepper to taste
- Fresh parsley for garnish

Preparation:

1. Heat olive oil in a large pot over medium heat.

2. Add onions, carrots, and celery, and sauté until softened.

3. Stir in lentils, vegetable broth, thyme, and bay leaf.

4. Bring to a boil, then reduce heat and simmer for 30 minutes, or until lentils are tender.

5. Season with salt and pepper.

6. Serve hot, garnished with fresh parsley.

Nutritional Values: (per serving)

- Calories: 180
- Protein: 11g
- Fat: 5g

- Carbohydrates: 25g
- Fiber: 10g

Cooking Time: 40 minutes

Serves: 4

Rating: ★★★★★

Seafood Chowder

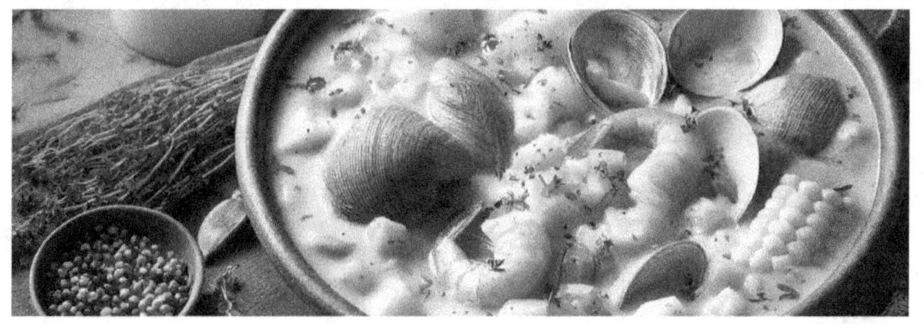

Ingredients:

- 1/2 lb shrimp, peeled and deveined
- 1/2 lb clams, cleaned
- 1/2 lb white fish, cubed
- 2 potatoes, diced
- 1 cup corn kernels
- 2 cups cream

- 4 cups chicken broth
- 1/2 cup white wine
- 1 teaspoon dried thyme
- 2 tablespoons olive oil
- Salt and pepper to taste
- Fresh parsley and oyster crackers for garnish

Preparation:

1. Heat olive oil in a large pot over medium heat.

2. Add potatoes and cook until slightly tender.

3. Pour in chicken broth and bring to a boil.

4. Add shrimp, clams, fish, corn, cream, white wine, and thyme.

5. Simmer until seafood is cooked through and potatoes are tender, about 20 minutes.

6. Season with salt and pepper.

7. Serve garnished with fresh parsley and oyster crackers.

Nutritional Values: (per serving)

- Calories: 400
- Protein: 25g
- Fat: 22g

- Carbohydrates: 20g
- Fiber: 2g

Cooking Time: 30 minutes

Serves: 4

Rating: ★★★★★

Tomato and Basil Soup

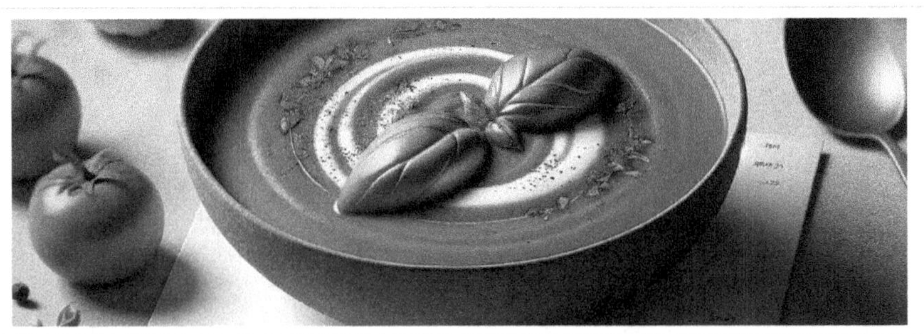

Ingredients:

- 4 cups ripe tomatoes, chopped
- 1 onion, chopped
- 2 cloves garlic, minced
- 1/4 cup fresh basil leaves
- 2 cups vegetable broth
- 1/2 cup cream
- 2 tablespoons olive oil
- Salt and pepper to taste

Preparation:

1. Heat olive oil in a large pot over medium heat.

2. Add onion and garlic, sauté until translucent.

3. Add tomatoes and cook until they break down and become soft.

4. Stir in vegetable broth and bring to a simmer.

5. Add basil leaves and simmer for 10 minutes.

6. Blend the soup until smooth.

7. Stir in cream, heat through. Season with salt and pepper.

8. Serve hot, garnished with a swirl of cream and fresh basil leaves.

Nutritional Values: (per serving)

- Calories: 200
- Protein: 3g
- Fat: 15g
- Carbohydrates: 15g
- Fiber: 3g

Cooking Time: 30 minutes

Serves: 4

Rating: ★★★★★

Desserts

Our dessert department has a delicious selection of sweet sweets that will fulfill your appetites without jeopardizing your health goals. These dishes strike a balance between indulgence and healthful ingredients, offering options that are both tasty and healthy. From fruit-based treats and rich, dark chocolate masterpieces to lighter variations of traditional favorites, each dessert is designed to bring joy and satisfaction. Whether you're searching for a fast sweet snack or a spectacular end to your meal, our desserts are ideal for guilt-free indulgence

Berry and Mascarpone Tart

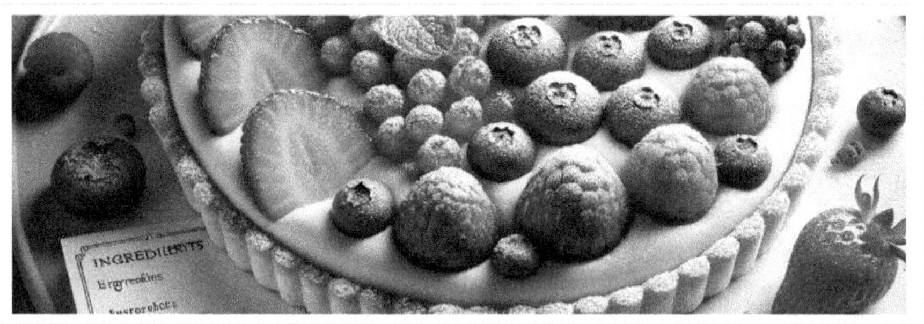

Ingredients:

- 1 prebaked pastry crust
- 1 cup mascarpone cheese

- 1/2 cup heavy cream
- 1/4 cup sugar

- 1 teaspoon vanilla extract
- 2 cups assorted fresh berries (strawberries, blueberries, raspberries)
- Powdered sugar for dusting
- Mint leaves for garnish

Preparation:

1. In a mixing bowl, whip mascarpone cheese, heavy cream, sugar, and vanilla extract until smooth and creamy.
2. Spread the mascarpone mixture into the prebaked pastry crust.
3. Arrange fresh berries on top of the filling.
4. Refrigerate for at least 2 hours to set.
5. Before serving, dust with powdered sugar and garnish with mint leaves.

Nutritional Values: (per serving)

- Calories: 350
- Protein: 4g
- Fat: 22g
- Carbohydrates: 34g
- Fiber: 2g

Cooking Time: 2 hours 20 minutes (including chilling)

Serves: 8

Rating: ★★★★★

Chocolate Avocado Pudding

Ingredients:

- 2 ripe avocados, peeled and pitted
- 1/4 cup cocoa powder

- 1/4 cup maple syrup
- 1 teaspoon vanilla extract
- Pinch of salt
- Dark chocolate shavings for garnish
- Fresh raspberries for garnish

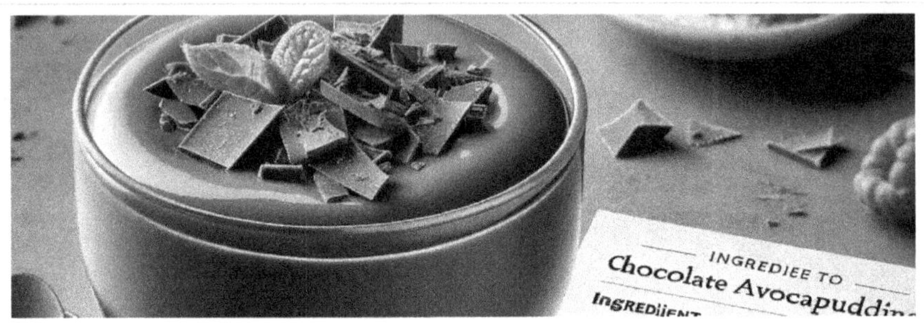

Preparation:

1. Combine avocados, cocoa powder, maple syrup, vanilla extract, and salt in a blender. Blend until smooth.
2. Transfer the mixture to serving bowls.
3. Chill in the refrigerator for at least 1 hour.
4. Garnish with dark chocolate shavings and fresh raspberries before serving.

Nutritional Values: (per serving)

- Calories: 240
- Protein: 3g
- Fat: 15g
- Carbohydrates: 28g
- Fiber: 7g

Cooking Time: 1 hour 10 minutes (including chilling)

Serves: 4

Rating: ★★★★★

Almond Flour Brownies

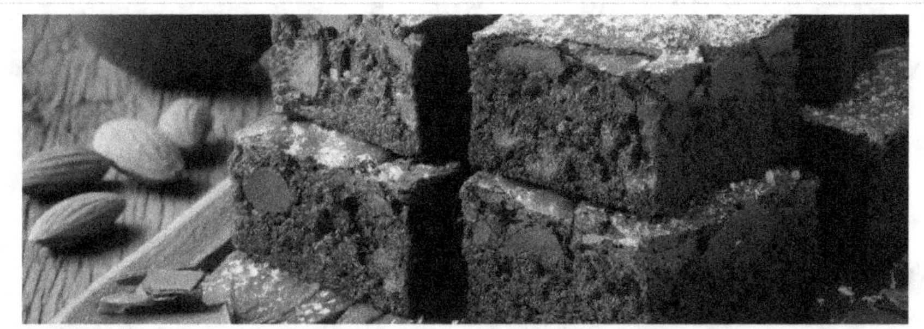

Ingredients:

- 2 cups almond flour
- 3/4 cup cocoa powder
- 3 eggs
- 1/2 cup coconut oil, melted
- 1 cup sugar
- 1 teaspoon vanilla extract
- 1 teaspoon baking powder
- 1/4 teaspoon salt
- 1/2 cup dark chocolate chunks
- Powdered sugar for dusting (optional)

Preparation:

1. Preheat the oven to 350°F (175°C).
2. In a bowl, mix almond flour, cocoa powder, baking powder, and salt.
3. In another bowl, whisk eggs, sugar, melted coconut oil, and vanilla extract.
4. Combine the wet and dry ingredients. Fold in dark chocolate chunks.

5. Pour the batter into a greased 8x8 inch baking pan.

6. Bake for 25-30 minutes or until a toothpick inserted comes out with few crumbs.

7. Let cool before cutting into squares. Dust with powdered sugar if desired.

Nutritional Values: (per serving)

- Calories: 280
- Protein: 6g
- Fat: 22g

- Carbohydrates: 21g
- Fiber: 3g

Cooking Time: 30 minutes

Serves: 12

Rating: ★★★★★

Coconut Flour Pancakes

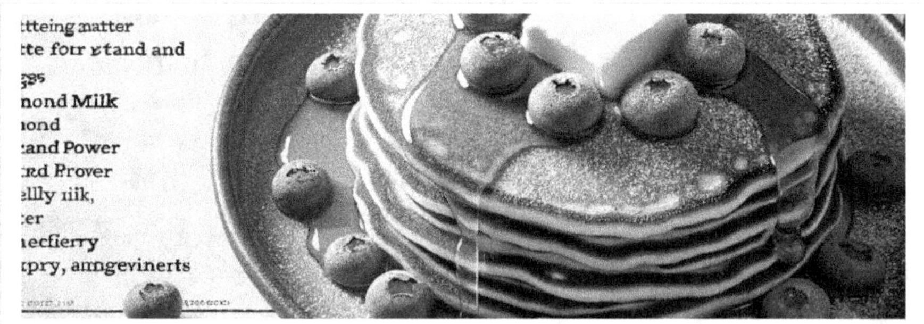

Ingredients:

- 1/2 cup coconut flour
- 4 eggs
- 1 cup almond milk

- 1 teaspoon baking powder
- 1 teaspoon vanilla extract
- Pinch of salt

- Butter for cooking
- Maple syrup and fresh blueberries for serving

Preparation:

1. In a bowl, whisk together coconut flour, baking powder, and salt.
2. In another bowl, beat eggs, almond milk, and vanilla extract until smooth.
3. Combine wet and dry ingredients to form a batter.
4. Heat butter in a skillet over medium heat. Pour batter to form pancakes.
5. Cook until golden on both sides, about 2-3 minutes per side.
6. Serve hot with maple syrup and fresh blueberries.

Nutritional Values: (per serving)

- Calories: 150
- Carbohydrates: 12g
- Protein: 6g
- Fiber: 3g
- Fat: 8g

Cooking Time: 15 minutes

Serves: 4

Rating: ★★★★★

Baked Apples with Cinnamon

Ingredients:

- 4 large apples, cored
- 1/4 cup raisins
- 1/2 cup oats
- 2 teaspoons cinnamon

- 2 tablespoons honey
- 1/2 cup water

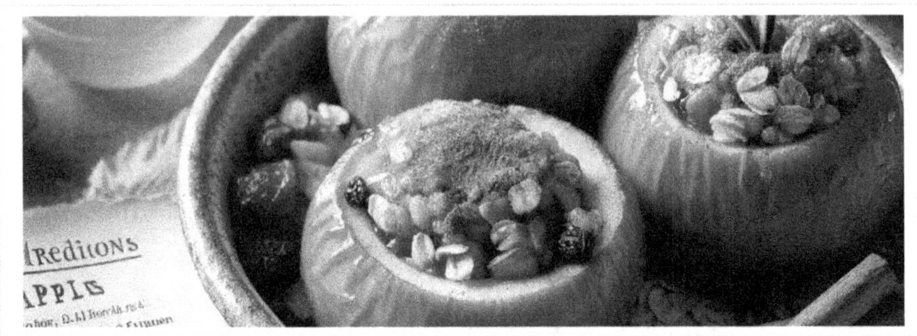

Preparation:

1. Preheat oven to 350°F (175°C).

2. Mix oats, raisins, and 1 teaspoon cinnamon.

3. Stuff the apples with the oat mixture and place them in a baking dish.

4. Drizzle honey over the apples and sprinkle with the remaining cinnamon.

5. Add water to the bottom of the dish.

6. Bake for 30-35 minutes, until the apples are tender.

7. Serve warm.

Nutritional Values: (per serving)

- Calories: 190
- Carbohydrates: 50g
- Protein: 1g
- Fiber: 6g
- Fat: 0.5g

Cooking Time: 35 minutes

Serves: 4

Rating: ★★★★★

Vegetarian and Vegan

Our Vegetarian & Vegan area is a bright celebration of plant-based eating, catering to people who choose a meatless lifestyle. These recipes highlight the richness and variety of vegetarian and vegan cuisine, ranging from robust dinners to light and refreshing salads. Each recipe is designed with health and flavor in mind, using only fresh, whole ingredients that provide both nutrition and delight. Whether you're a lifelong vegetarian, a dedicated vegan, or simply trying to add more plant-based meals into your diet, this section contains a wide range of foods that will inspire and please you at every meal

Tofu Stir-Fry

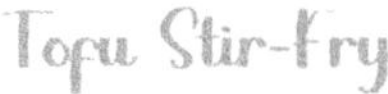

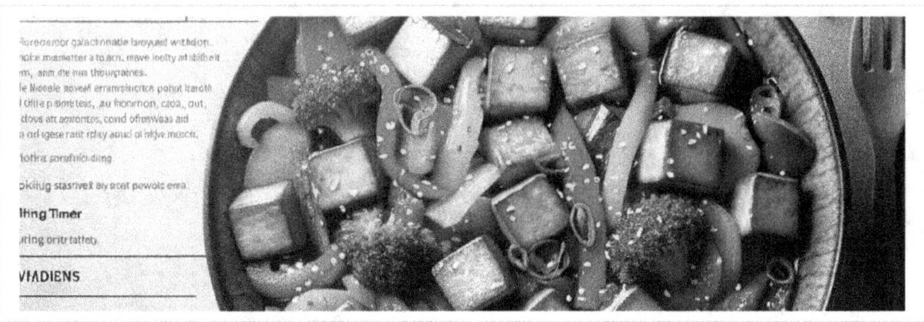

Ingredients:

- 1 lb tofu, pressed and cubed

- 1 bell pepper, sliced

- 1 cup broccoli florets
- 1 carrot, sliced
- 2 tablespoons soy sauce
- 1 tablespoon sesame oil
- 2 cloves garlic, minced
- 1 inch ginger, minced
- Sesame seeds for garnish
- Green onions, sliced for garnish

Preparation:

1. Heat sesame oil in a large skillet over medium-high heat.
2. Add garlic and ginger, sauté for 1 minute.
3. Add tofu and cook until golden on all sides.
4. Add bell pepper, broccoli, and carrot. Stir-fry for about 5 minutes.
5. Stir in soy sauce and cook for another 2 minutes.
6. Garnish with sesame seeds and green onions.

Nutritional Values: (per serving)

- Calories: 200
- Protein: 12g
- Fat: 12g
- Carbohydrates: 10g
- Fiber: 3g

Cooking Time: 15 minutes

Serves: 4

Rating: ★★★★★

Veggie Burger

Ingredients:

- 1 cup cooked black beans
- 1/2 cup cooked quinoa
- 1/2 cup finely chopped vegetables (carrots, onions, bell peppers)
- Whole wheat buns
- Lettuce leaves

- Tomato slices
- Avocado slices
- Vegan mayo
- Spices (cumin, paprika)
- Salt and pepper

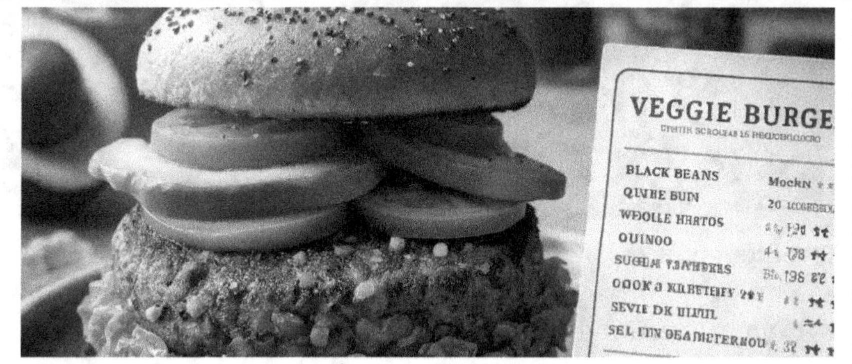

Preparation:

1. Mash black beans in a bowl. Mix in quinoa, chopped vegetables, spices, salt, and pepper.
2. Form the mixture into patties.
3. Grill the patties until heated through and crispy on the outside.
4. Assemble the burgers on whole wheat buns with lettuce, tomato, avocado, and a dollop of vegan mayo.

Nutritional Values: (per serving)

- Calories: 320

- Protein: 10g

- Fat: 9g
- Carbohydrates: 45g
- Fiber: 10g

Cooking Time: 20 minutes

Serves: 4

Rating: ★★★★★

Mushroom Stroganoff

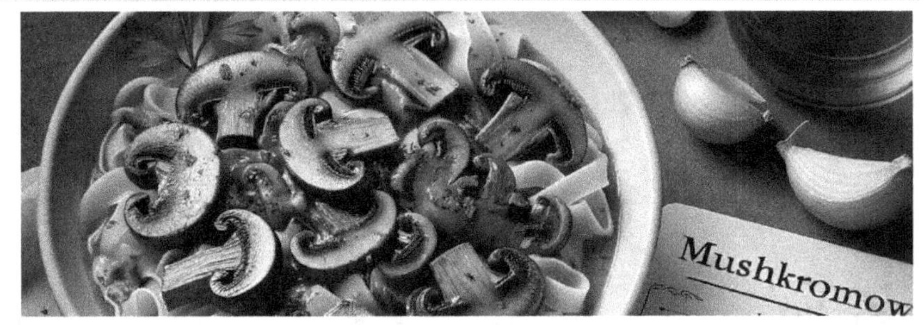

Ingredients:

- 1 lb mixed mushrooms (such as portobello and cremini), sliced
- 1 large onion, chopped
- 2 cloves garlic, minced
- 2 cups vegetable broth
- 1 cup sour cream
- 8 oz egg noodles
- 2 tablespoons olive oil
- Salt and pepper to taste
- Fresh parsley, chopped for garnish

Preparation:

1. Heat olive oil in a large skillet over medium heat.
2. Add onions and garlic, sauté until translucent.

3. Add mushrooms and cook until they release their juices and begin to brown.

4. Pour in vegetable broth and bring to a simmer.

5. Stir in sour cream and season with salt and pepper. Simmer until the sauce thickens slightly.

6. Cook egg noodles according to package instructions.

7. Serve stroganoff over noodles, garnished with chopped parsley.

Nutritional Values: (per serving)

- Calories: 400
- Protein: 14g
- Fat: 20g
- Carbohydrates: 45g
- Fiber: 5g

Cooking Time: 30 minutes

Serves: 4

Rating: ★★★★★

Vegan Chili

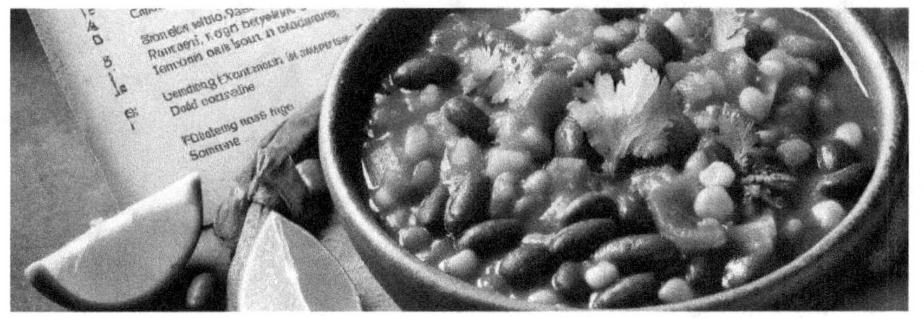

Ingredients:

- 1 can kidney beans, drained and rinsed
- 1 can black beans, drained and rinsed
- 1 can pinto beans, drained and rinsed
- 1 cup corn kernels
- 1 red bell pepper, chopped
- 1 green bell pepper, chopped
- 1 onion, chopped
- 2 cloves garlic, minced
- 1 can diced tomatoes
- 2 cups tomato sauce
- 1 teaspoon cumin
- 1 teaspoon chili powder
- 1/2 teaspoon smoked paprika
- 2 tablespoons olive oil
- Salt and pepper to taste
- Avocado, sliced for garnish
- Cilantro, chopped for garnish
- Lime wedges for serving

Preparation:

1. Heat olive oil in a large pot over medium heat.
2. Add onions, garlic, and bell peppers, sauté until soft.
3. Stir in all beans, corn, diced tomatoes, and tomato sauce.
4. Season with cumin, chili powder, and smoked paprika.
5. Simmer for 30 minutes, stirring occasionally.
6. Serve hot, garnished with avocado slices, chopped cilantro, and a lime wedge.

Nutritional Values: (per serving)

- Calories: 320
- Protein: 15g

- Fat: 8g
- Carbohydrates: 50g

- Fiber: 15g

Cooking Time: 40 minutes

Serves: 6

Rating: ★★★★★

Stuffed Bell Peppers

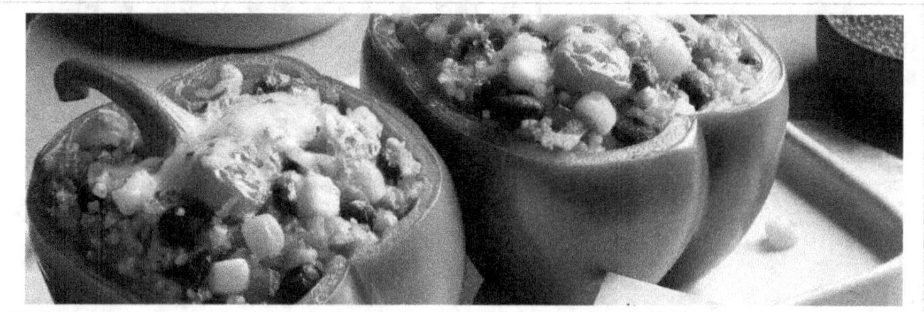

Ingredients:

- 4 large bell peppers, tops cut off and seeds removed
- 1 cup cooked quinoa
- 1 can black beans, drained and rinsed
- 1 cup corn kernels
- 1 can diced tomatoes, drained

- 1 cup shredded cheese
- 2 tablespoons olive oil
- 1 teaspoon cumin
- 1 teaspoon chili powder
- Salt and pepper to taste

Preparation:

1. Preheat oven to 375°F (190°C).

2. In a bowl, mix quinoa, black beans, corn, diced tomatoes, cumin, chili powder, salt, and pepper.

3. Stuff each bell pepper with the quinoa mixture and place in a baking dish.

4. Drizzle with olive oil and cover with foil.

5. Bake for 30 minutes, then remove foil, top with cheese, and bake for another 10 minutes until the cheese is melted and bubbly.

6. Serve hot.

Nutritional Values: (per serving)

- Calories: 350
- Protein: 15g
- Fat: 12g
- Carbohydrates: 45g
- Fiber: 9g

Cooking Time: 40 minutes

Serves: 4

Rating: ★★★★★

Butternut Squash Soup

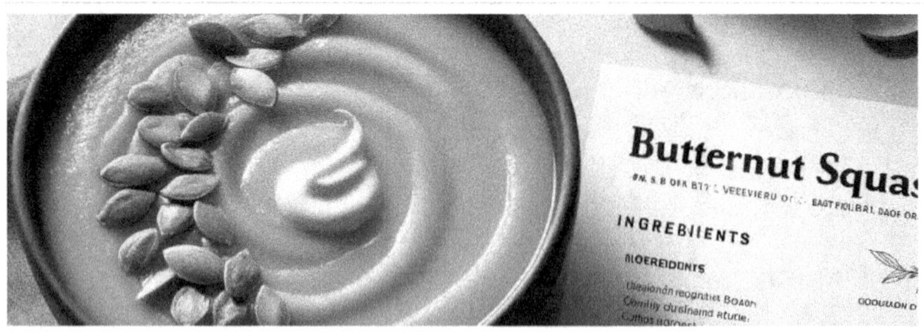

Ingredients:

- 1 large butternut squash, peeled and cubed
- 1 onion, chopped
- 2 cloves garlic, minced
- 4 cups vegetable broth
- 1/2 cup cream
- 2 tablespoons olive oil
- Salt and pepper to taste
- Pumpkin seeds, toasted for garnish

Preparation:

1. Heat olive oil in a large pot over medium heat.
2. Add onion and garlic, sauté until soft.
3. Add butternut squash and vegetable broth, bring to a boil.
4. Reduce heat and simmer until squash is tender, about 20 minutes.
5. Puree the soup in a blender or with an immersion blender until smooth.
6. Stir in cream, season with salt and pepper.
7. Serve hot, garnished with a swirl of cream and toasted pumpkin seeds.

Nutritional Values: (per serving)

- Calories: 200
- Protein: 3g
- Fat: 12g
- Carbohydrates: 22g
- Fiber: 5g

Cooking Time: 35 minutes

Serves: 4

Rating: ★★★★★

Vegan Tacos

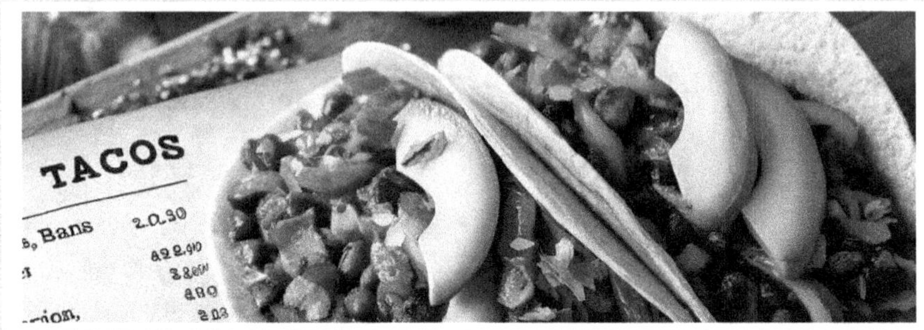

Ingredients:

- 1 can black beans, drained and rinsed
- 1 bell pepper, sliced
- 1 onion, sliced
- 1 avocado, sliced
- 1/4 cup chopped cilantro
- Juice of 1 lime
- 1 cup shredded cabbage
- 8 corn tortillas
- 2 tablespoons olive oil
- 1 teaspoon cumin
- 1 teaspoon chili powder
- Salt and pepper to taste

Preparation:

1. Heat olive oil in a skillet over medium heat.
2. Add onions and bell peppers, sauté until softened.
3. Stir in black beans, cumin, and chili powder, cook until heated through.
4. Warm tortillas on a skillet or in the microwave.
5. Assemble tacos with the bean mixture, avocado slices, and cabbage slaw mixed with cilantro and lime juice.

6. Serve immediately.

Nutritional Values: (per serving)

- Calories: 280
- Protein: 8g
- Fat: 10g

- Carbohydrates: 40g
- Fiber: 10g

Cooking Time: 20 minutes

Serves: 4

Ratin: ★★★★★

Lentil Salad

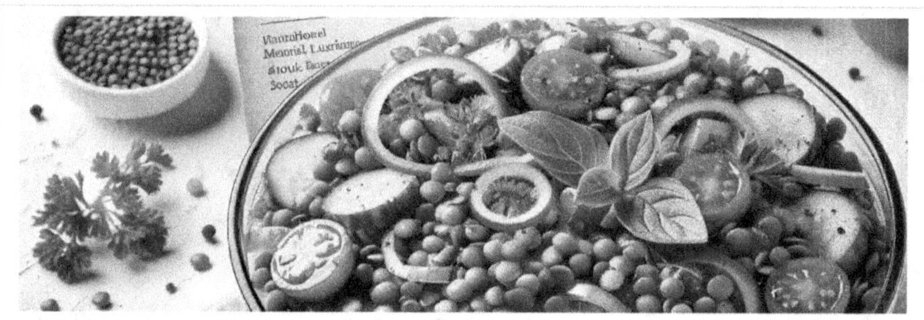

Ingredients:

- 1 cup green lentils, cooked
- 1 cucumber, diced
- 1 cup cherry tomatoes, halved
- 1/2 red onion, finely chopped

- 1/4 cup chopped parsley
- 3 tablespoons olive oil
- Juice of 1 lemon
- 1 clove garlic, minced
- Salt and pepper to taste

Preparation:

1. In a large bowl, combine cooked lentils, cucumber, cherry tomatoes, red onion, and parsley.

2. In a small bowl, whisk together olive oil, lemon juice, garlic, salt, and pepper to make the dressing.

3. Pour the dressing over the salad and toss to combine.

4. Chill in the refrigerator before serving to enhance the flavors.

Nutritional Values: (per serving)

- Calories: 200
- Protein: 10g
- Fat: 7g
- Carbohydrates: 28g
- Fiber: 8g

Cooking Time: 10 minutes (plus chilling)

Serves: 4   **Rating:** ★★★★★

Spinach and Mushroom Quiche

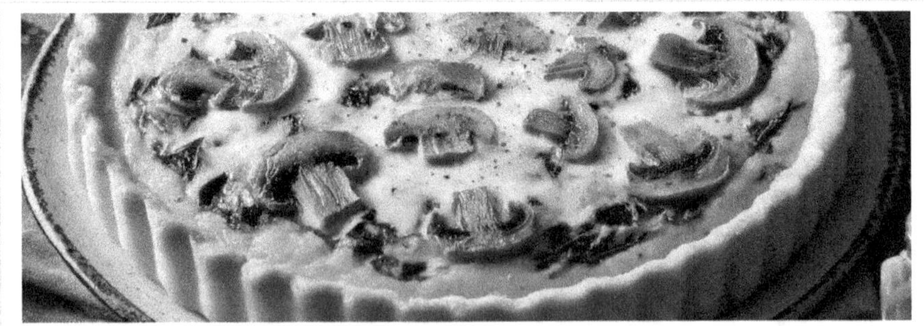

Ingredients:

- 1 prebaked pie crust
- 4 eggs
- 1 cup cream

- 1 cup fresh spinach, chopped
- 1 cup mushrooms, sliced
- 1/2 cup grated cheese
- 2 tablespoons olive oil
- Salt and pepper to taste

Preparation:

1. Preheat oven to 375°F (190°C).
2. Heat olive oil in a skillet over medium heat. Sauté mushrooms until they are soft, about 5 minutes.
3. Add spinach to the skillet and cook until wilted.
4. In a bowl, whisk together eggs and cream. Season with salt and pepper.
5. Stir in the sautéed mushrooms and spinach.
6. Pour the egg mixture into the pie crust and sprinkle with grated cheese.
7. Bake for 30-35 minutes or until the center is set and the top is golden.
8. Let cool slightly before serving.

Nutritional Values: (per serving)

- Calories: 350
- Protein: 12g
- Fat: 28g
- Carbohydrates: 12g
- Fiber: 1g

Cooking Time: 45 minutes

Serves: 6

Rating: ★★★★★

Vegetable Curry

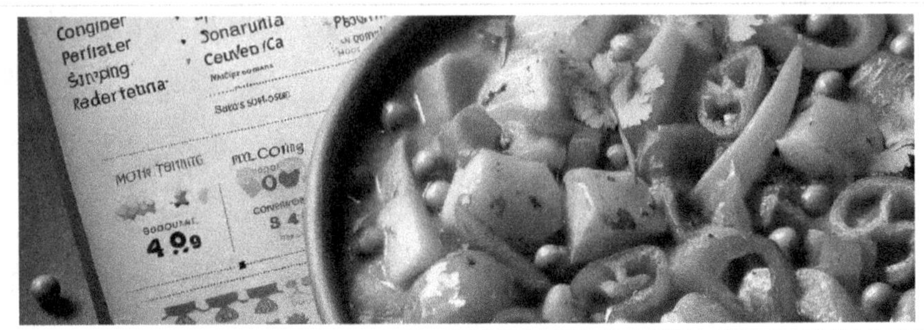

Ingredients:

- 1 bell pepper, chopped
- 2 carrots, sliced
- 2 potatoes, cubed
- 1 cup peas
- 1 can coconut milk
- 2 tablespoons curry powder
- 2 cloves garlic, minced
- 1 inch ginger, minced
- 1 onion, chopped
- 2 tablespoons olive oil
- Salt and pepper to taste
- Fresh cilantro and red chili slices for garnish

Preparation:

1. Heat olive oil in a large pot over medium heat.
2. Add onion, garlic, and ginger, sauté until fragrant.
3. Stir in carrots, potatoes, bell pepper, and curry powder. Cook for about 5 minutes.
4. Pour in coconut milk and bring to a simmer.
5. Add peas and cook until all vegetables are tender, about 20 minutes.

6. Season with salt and pepper.

7. Garnish with cilantro and red chili slices before serving.

Nutritional Values: (per serving)

- Calories: 250
- Protein: 5g
- Fat: 18g
- Carbohydrates: 20g
- Fiber: 5g

Cooking Time: 30 minutes

Serves: 4

Rating: ★★★★★

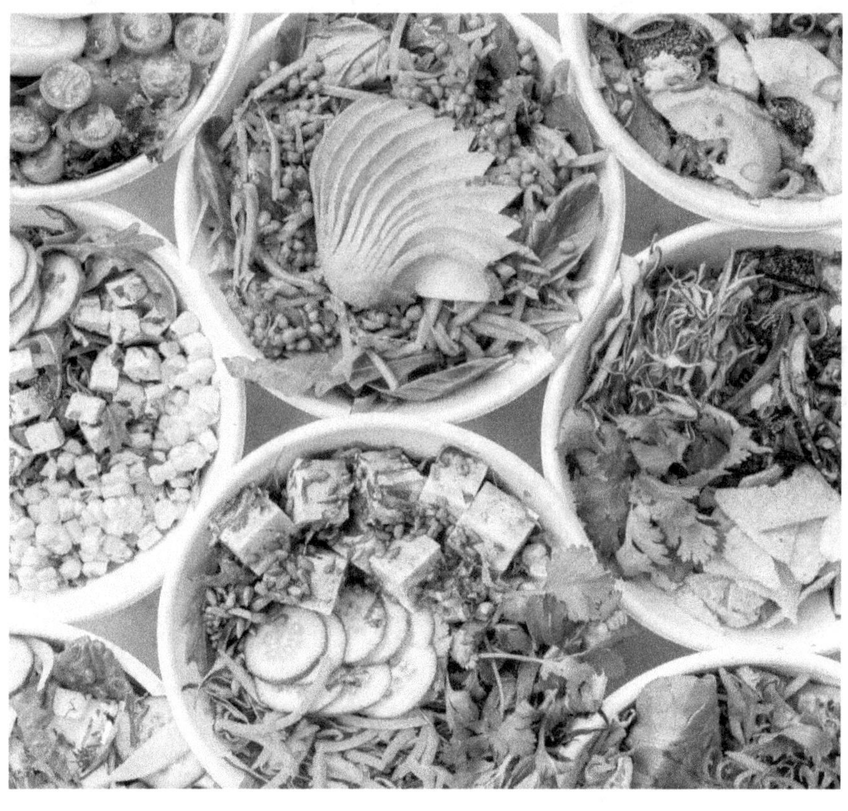

Condiments, Dressings, and Sauces

Explore our condiments, dressings, and sauces, all of which are designed to add vibrant flavors and textures to any cuisine. This area has a wide variety of recipes, from rich, creamy dressings to zesty, herb-infused sauces that can elevate simple meals into exceptional experiences. Whether spreading over a salad, complementing a grilled dish, or adding depth to a stew, these expertly designed recipes use fresh, healthful ingredients to enhance any meal. Perfect for those wishing to add some innovation to their culinary arsenal, each recipe is not only delicious but also simple to prepare, allowing you to introduce new flavors to your table with ease.

Avocado Lime Dressing

Ingredients:

- 1 ripe avocado, peeled and pitted
- Juice of 2 limes
- 1/4 cup olive oil
- 1 clove garlic, minced
- 1/4 cup fresh cilantro, chopped
- Salt and pepper to taste
- Water to thin (optional)

Preparation:

1. In a blender or food processor, combine the avocado, lime juice, olive oil, garlic, and cilantro.
2. Blend until smooth.
3. Season with salt and pepper to taste.
4. If the dressing is too thick, add water a tablespoon at a time until desired consistency is reached.
5. Serve over salads, grilled vegetables, or use as a dip.

Nutritional Values: (approximation per serving)

- Calories: 100
- Protein: 1g
- Fat: 10g

- Carbohydrates: 4g
- Fiber: 2g

Serves: Makes about 1 cup

Rating: ★★★★★

This creamy and tangy dressing brings a burst of freshness to any dish, enhancing flavors with its rich and smooth texture.

Tomato Basil Sauce

Ingredients:

- 2 cans (14.5 oz each) diced tomatoes
- 1 onion, finely chopped
- 3 cloves garlic, minced
- 1/4 cup fresh basil leaves, chopped

- 2 tablespoons olive oil
- 1 teaspoon sugar (optional, to balance acidity)
- Salt and pepper to taste

Preparation:

1. Heat olive oil in a saucepan over medium heat.

2. Add the chopped onion and garlic, sauté until they are soft and translucent.

3. Pour in the diced tomatoes, including the juice.

4. Simmer the mixture for 20 minutes, allowing the flavors to meld together.

5. Add the chopped basil, sugar (if using), and season with salt and pepper.

6. Cook for an additional 10 minutes.

7. Use an immersion blender to blend the sauce slightly, if a smoother consistency is desired.

8. Serve over pasta, as a base for pizzas, or with your favorite meatballs.

Nutritional Values: (approximation per serving)

- Calories: 70
- Protein: 1g
- Fat: 5g
- Carbohydrates: 6g
- Fiber: 1g

Serves: 4   **Rating:** ★★★★★

This simple yet flavorful sauce captures the essence of fresh tomatoes and basil, perfect for enhancing any Italian dish.

Peanut Sauce

Ingredients:

- 1/2 cup smooth peanut butter
- 1/4 cup soy sauce
- 2 tablespoons lime juice
- 2 tablespoons honey or brown sugar
- 1 clove garlic, minced
- 1 teaspoon grated ginger
- 1/4 teaspoon chili flakes (adjust to taste)
- 1/2 cup warm water (adjust for desired consistency)

Preparation:

1. In a bowl, combine peanut butter, soy sauce, lime juice, honey or sugar, garlic, ginger, and chili flakes.
2. Gradually whisk in warm water until the sauce reaches your preferred consistency. It should be smooth and pourable.
3. Taste and adjust seasoning as needed, adding more lime juice for acidity, honey for sweetness, or chili flakes for heat.

Nutritional Values: (approximation per serving)

- Calories: 150
- Protein: 4g
- Fat: 10g
- Carbohydrates: 12g
- Fiber: 1g

Serves: Makes about 1 cup

Rating: ★★★★★

This versatile peanut sauce is perfect for drizzling over salads, using as a dip for spring rolls, or as a flavorful addition to stir-fries and noodles. Its rich, creamy texture and balance of sweet, savory, and spicy flavors make it a crowd-pleaser.

Cilantro Lime Vinaigrette

Ingredients:

- Juice of 2 limes
- 1/3 cup olive oil
- 1/4 cup fresh cilantro, finely chopped
- 1 clove garlic, minced
- 1 tablespoon honey
- Salt and pepper to taste

Preparation:

1. In a small bowl or jar, combine the lime juice, olive oil, chopped cilantro, minced garlic, and honey.
2. Whisk together until well blended or shake vigorously if using a jar.
3. Season with salt and pepper according to your taste preferences.
4. Let the vinaigrette sit for at least 10 minutes before serving to allow the flavors to meld together.
5. Drizzle over fresh salads, grilled vegetables, or use as a marinade for chicken or fish.

Nutritional Values: (approximation per serving)

- Calories: 100
- Protein: 0g

- Fat: 9g
- Carbohydrates: 4g

- Fiber: 0g

Serves: Makes about 1/2 cup

Rating: ★★★★★

This Cilantro Lime Vinaigrette is a vibrant and tangy dressing that enhances the flavors of any dish, adding a fresh zesty note with a hint of sweetness.

Creamy Garlic Aioli

Ingredients:

- 1 cup mayonnaise
- 3 cloves garlic, minced
- 2 tablespoons lemon juice
-

- 1 teaspoon Dijon mustard
- Salt and pepper to taste

Preparation:

1. In a small bowl, combine mayonnaise, minced garlic, lemon juice, and Dijon mustard.
2. Whisk together until the mixture is smooth and well-blended.
3. Season with salt and pepper according to your taste preferences.
4. Cover and refrigerate for at least 30 minutes before serving to allow the flavors to meld together.
5. Serve as a dip for vegetables, a spread for sandwiches, or a topping for grilled meats.

Nutritional Values: (approximation per serving)

- Calories: 100 (per tablespoon)
- Protein: 0g
- Fat: 10g
- Carbohydrates: 1g
- Fiber: 0g

Serves: Makes about 1 cup

Rating: ★★★★★

This Creamy Garlic Aioli is a rich and flavorful condiment that adds a luxurious touch to simple dishes, providing a smooth, garlicky complement that enhances flavors beautifully.

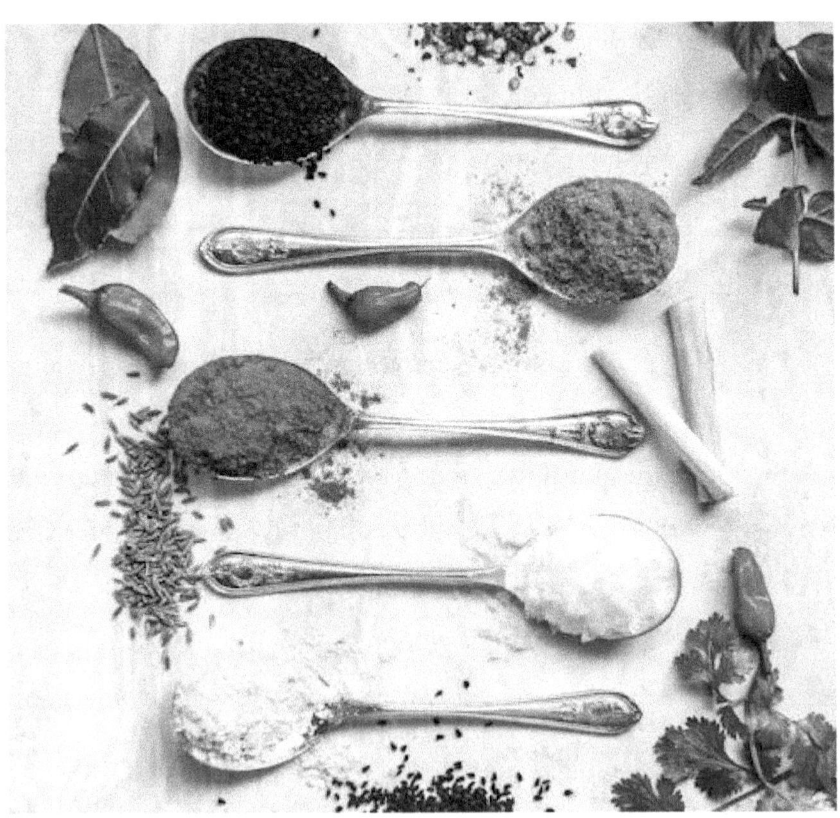

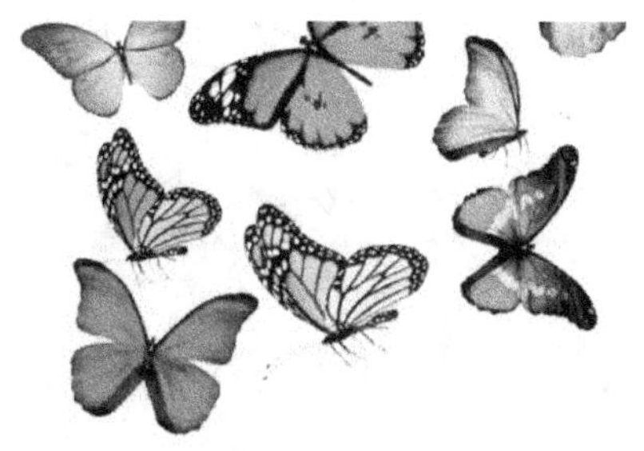

Part 4: Living with Insulin Resistance

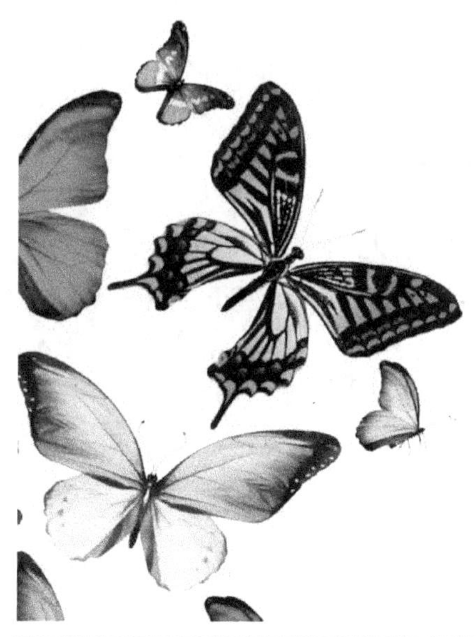

7-Day Sample Meal Planning and Prep for Busy Lives

Our meal planning guide is designed to simplify your weekly cooking while maintaining a balanced and delicious diet. Using the recipes provided in our cookbook, this 7-day sample menu integrates various dishes, emphasizing ease of preparation and nutrient diversity. Each day combines different flavors and ingredients, ensuring that meals remain exciting and healthful.

Meal Preparation Tips:

1. **Batch Cooking:** Cook staples like quinoa, rice, and beans in large quantities to use throughout the week.

2. **Prep Vegetables:** Wash, chop, and store vegetables in the refrigerator to save time on busy days.

3. **Pre-make Sauces and Dressings:** Prepare any sauces and dressings ahead of time and store them in the refrigerator.

4. **Plan for Leftovers:** Use leftovers creatively in salads, wraps, or as ingredients in other recipes to minimize waste.

7-Day Sample Meal Plan

Day 1:

- **Breakfast:** Spinach and Feta Omelet

- **Lunch:** Chickpea and Avocado Salad

- **Dinner:** Chicken and Vegetable Stew

- **Snack:** Greek Yogurt with Berries

Day 2:

- **Breakfast:** Almond and Berry Smoothie

- **Lunch:** Turkey and Spinach Wrap

- **Dinner:** Beef Chili

- **Snack:** Kale Chips

Day 3:

- **Breakfast:** Quinoa Breakfast Bowl

- **Lunch:** Quinoa and Black Bean Bowl

- **Dinner:** Grilled Salmon with Asparagus

- **Snack:** Avocado Chocolate Mousse

Day 4:

- **Breakfast:** Protein Pancakes

- **Lunch:** Grilled Vegetable Platter

- **Dinner:** Mushroom Stroganoff

- **Snack:** Cucumber and Hummus Bites

Day 5:

- **Breakfast:** Avocado Toast with Poached Egg

- **Lunch:** Tuna Salad Stuffed Avocados

- **Dinner:** Eggplant Lasagna

- **Snack:** Almonds and Cheese

Day 6:

- **Breakfast:** Overnight Oats with Nuts

- **Lunch:** Lentil Soup

- **Dinner:** Pork Tenderloin with Roasted Vegetables

- **Snack:** Peanut Sauce with Veggies

Day 7:

- **Breakfast:** Breakfast Tacos with Cauliflower Tortilla

- **Lunch:** Veggie Burger

- **Dinner:** Vegan Tacos

- **Snack:** Berry and Mascarpone Tart

Shopping List: To make shopping more manageable, compile a list based on the meal plan, categorizing items by produce, dairy, pantry staples, and meats. Ensure to check what items you already have to avoid duplicate purchases.

Preparation Steps:

- **Sunday Prep:** Cook grains like quinoa and prepare proteins such as chicken or turkey for use in meals. Wash and chop vegetables.

- **Midweek Prep:** Reassess what's left and prepare additional items if needed. This can include more vegetables or another batch of a staple like rice or pasta.

This structured plan not only simplifies the cooking process throughout the week but also ensures you enjoy a variety of flavors and nutrients. Happy eating!

Shopping List and Pantry Staples

To make your meal preparation efficient and enjoyable, having a well-stocked pantry and a detailed shopping list based on the weekly meal plan is crucial. Here's a breakdown to help guide your shopping for the week.

Produce:

- Spinach
- Berries (strawberries, blueberries, raspberries)
- Avocados
- Tomatoes (cherry and regular)
- Lettuce
- Cucumbers
- Carrots
- Bell peppers (various colors)
- Onions (red and white)
- Garlic
- Potatoes
- Fresh herbs (cilantro, parsley, basil)
- Lemons and limes
- Broccoli
- Cauliflower
- Mushrooms
- Zucchini
- Asparagus
- Eggplant
- Corn
- Green beans

Proteins:

- Eggs
- Chicken breast
- Ground beef
- Salmon fillets
- Turkey breast
- Pork tenderloin
- Canned black beans, chickpeas, and kidney beans
- Tofu

Dairy and Alternatives:

- Greek yogurt
- Feta cheese
- Cheddar cheese
- Sour cream

- Mascarpone cheese

- Vegan cheese (if preferred)

- Almond milk

Grains and Nuts:

- Quinoa

- Almond flour

- Oats

- Whole wheat bread and tortillas

- Corn tortillas

- Brown rice

- Almonds

- Coconut flour

Canned and Jarred Goods:

- Diced tomatoes

- Coconut milk

- Tomato sauce

- Peanut butter

Condiments and Spices:

- Olive oil

- Sesame oil

- Vinegar (balsamic, apple cider)

- Soy sauce

- Honey

- Maple syrup

- Salt and pepper

- Variety of dried herbs and spices (cumin, chili powder, smoked paprika, cinnamon, nutmeg)

- Vanilla extract

Pantry Staples:

- Baking powder

- Cocoa powder

- Sugar

- Nutritional yeast

- Flour (for those not gluten-sensitive)

Snacks and Others:

- Dark chocolate

- Pumpkin seeds

- Sesame seeds

- Popcorn (for healthy snacking)

Freezer Items:

- Frozen berries

- Frozen peas

This comprehensive list ensures you have a wide variety of ingredients that can be mixed and matched to create not only the recipes planned for the week but also allow for flexibility and creativity in your cooking. Adjust quantities based on your household size and dietary preferences.

Substitution Guide for Common Ingredients

Creating delicious meals even when you're missing an ingredient is all about smart substitutions. Here's a guide to help you replace common ingredients from the recipes in our book, ensuring you can still enjoy your meals without a last-minute store run.

Dairy and Dairy Alternatives:

- **Mascarpone Cheese:** Use cream cheese or a blend of cream cheese and heavy cream.

- **Greek Yogurt:** Substitute with sour cream or a non-dairy yogurt if vegan.

- **Sour Cream:** Use plain yogurt or crème fraîche.

Proteins:

- **Chicken Breast:** Replace with turkey breast or tofu for a vegetarian option.

- **Salmon Fillets:** Use trout or mackerel. For a vegetarian option, use thick slices of marinated and grilled eggplant.

- **Eggs:** For baking, use applesauce or mashed bananas (1/4 cup per egg). For cooking, try a tofu scramble.

Vegetables:

- **Spinach:** Substitute with kale or Swiss chard.

- **Mushrooms:** Try using zucchini or eggplant for a similar texture.

- **Bell Peppers:** Use carrots or celery for crunch in salads and stir-fries.

Grains:

- **Quinoa:** Replace with couscous or rice.

- **Almond Flour:** Use coconut flour or another nut flour.

- **Whole Wheat Bread:** Substitute with any whole grain bread or gluten-free bread if needed.

Fats and Oils:

- **Olive Oil:** Use avocado oil or canola oil.

- **Butter:** Use margarine or coconut oil for baking. For cooking, use olive oil or vegetable oil.

Condiments and Sauces:

- **Soy Sauce:** Use tamari or coconut aminos for a soy-free or gluten-free alternative.

- **Vinegar:** Almost any vinegar (except balsamic) can be substituted for another with slight taste differences.

- **Honey:** Replace with maple syrup or agave nectar.

Spices and Herbs:

- **Cilantro:** Use parsley or a mix of parsley and mint.

- **Cumin:** Ground coriander or a mix of ground caraway and oregano can provide a similar flavor profile.

- **Basil:** Try oregano or thyme for a different but complementary flavor.

Sweeteners:

- **Sugar:** Use honey, maple syrup, or agave nectar. For a non-caloric option, try stevia or erythritol.

Nuts and Seeds:

- **Almonds:** Use walnuts, pecans, or any other nut. For a nut-free option, try sunflower seeds or pumpkin seeds.

This substitution guide is intended to be flexible and adaptable to what you have on hand, helping you maintain the flavor and integrity of your meals while accommodating dietary preferences and ingredient availability.

Navigating Social Situations and Eating Out

Eating out and attending social gatherings can often present challenges, especially when you're trying to adhere to specific dietary preferences or restrictions. However, with a little planning and communication, you can enjoy these occasions without compromising your dietary goals. Here are some tips and strategies from our book to help you navigate social situations and dining out successfully:

1. Research Restaurants Ahead of Time:

- Before dining out, look up the restaurant's menu online. Many places now offer a variety of dietary options and list ingredients. Call ahead to discuss any dietary restrictions with the staff—they can often accommodate special requests if given notice.

2. Be Clear About Your Dietary Needs:

- Don't hesitate to clearly communicate your dietary needs to the waiter or chef. Being specific about what you can and cannot eat helps prevent any misunderstandings and ensures a more enjoyable meal.

3. Choose Wisely:

- Opt for dishes that are likely to fit within your dietary guidelines. Salads, grilled meats, and vegetable-based dishes are often safe bets. Be cautious of sauces and dressings, as they can contain hidden sugars and fats.

4. Plan for Social Gatherings:

- If you're attending a party or an event, consider eating a small, healthy meal beforehand so you won't be hungry if options are limited. Alternatively, offer to bring a dish to share that meets your dietary needs.

5. Learn to Politely Decline:

- If offered something that doesn't meet your dietary needs, politely decline. You can briefly explain your dietary restrictions, but a simple "No, thank you" is also perfectly acceptable.

6. Focus on Social Interaction:

- Shift the focus from food to enjoying the company of others. Engaging in conversations and participating in activities can take the emphasis off eating.

7. Enjoy Mindfully:

- When you do choose to indulge, do so mindfully. Savor the flavors and enjoy the experience, which can help prevent overeating and make the meal more satisfying.

8. Carry Snacks:

- Have a healthy snack before you go out, or bring one with you to avoid being tempted by unhealthy options.

By employing these strategies, you can enjoy social situations without stress and maintain your healthy eating habits even when you're not at home. This approach allows you to be flexible and accommodating to your social life, ensuring that your dietary preferences don't keep you from enjoying good times with family and friends.

Thank You

I'm writing this with a heart full of gratitude for your kind words and the time you took to read my book, knowing that my words have resonated with you is a reward beyond measure. Thank you again for your appreciation and for being a part of this literary journey.

Warmly,

Joan

For further Questions and advice reach out on

joanmilonehelpdesk@gmail.com

Your voice matters to us! Dive into the pages of our latest book and embark on a journey of discovery, adventure, and insight. Once you've turned the last page, we invite you to share your thoughts with us.

Your honest review is incredibly important for several reasons: It not only helps us grow and improve by understanding what resonates with our readers, but it also assists fellow readers in making informed decisions about their next reading choice. In a way, your feedback lights the path for future stories and enriches our reading community. So, take a moment, reflect on your journey through our story, and leave a review that could light the way for others. Together, let's create a community of passionate readers and insightful feedback.

Thank you for being a part of our story – we can't wait to hear from you!

Kindly open your phone camera and place it on the barcode to scan

It will link you directly to author page to access more cookbooks from us

Very seamless…

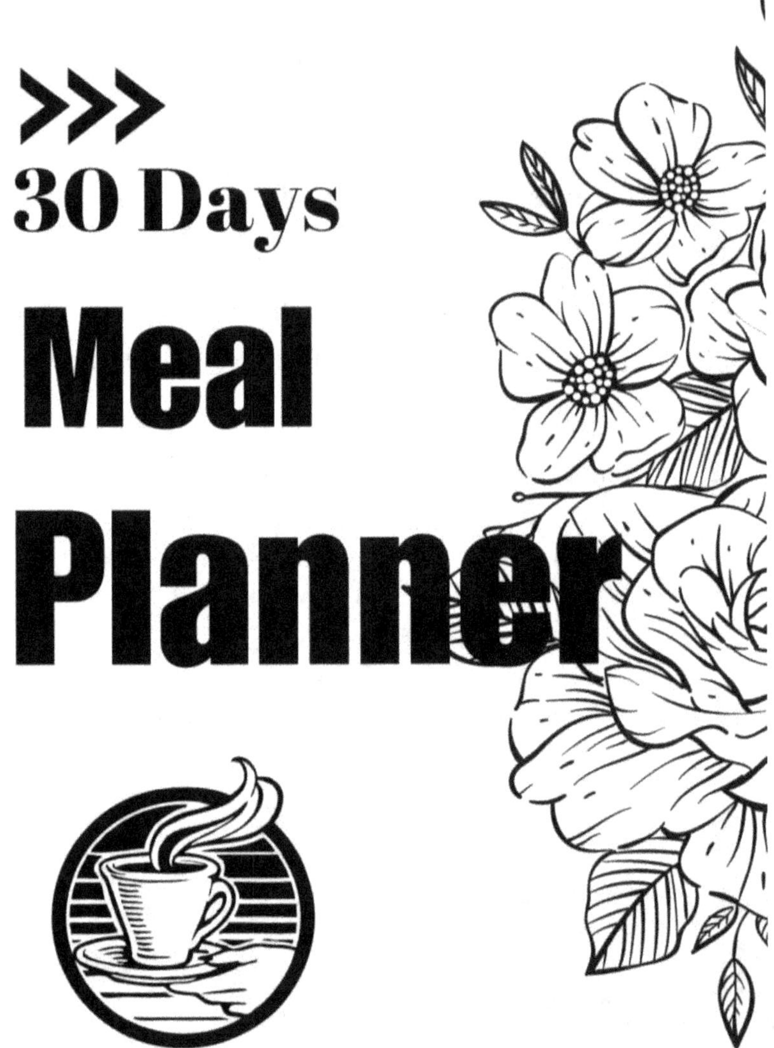
30 Days
Meal
Planner

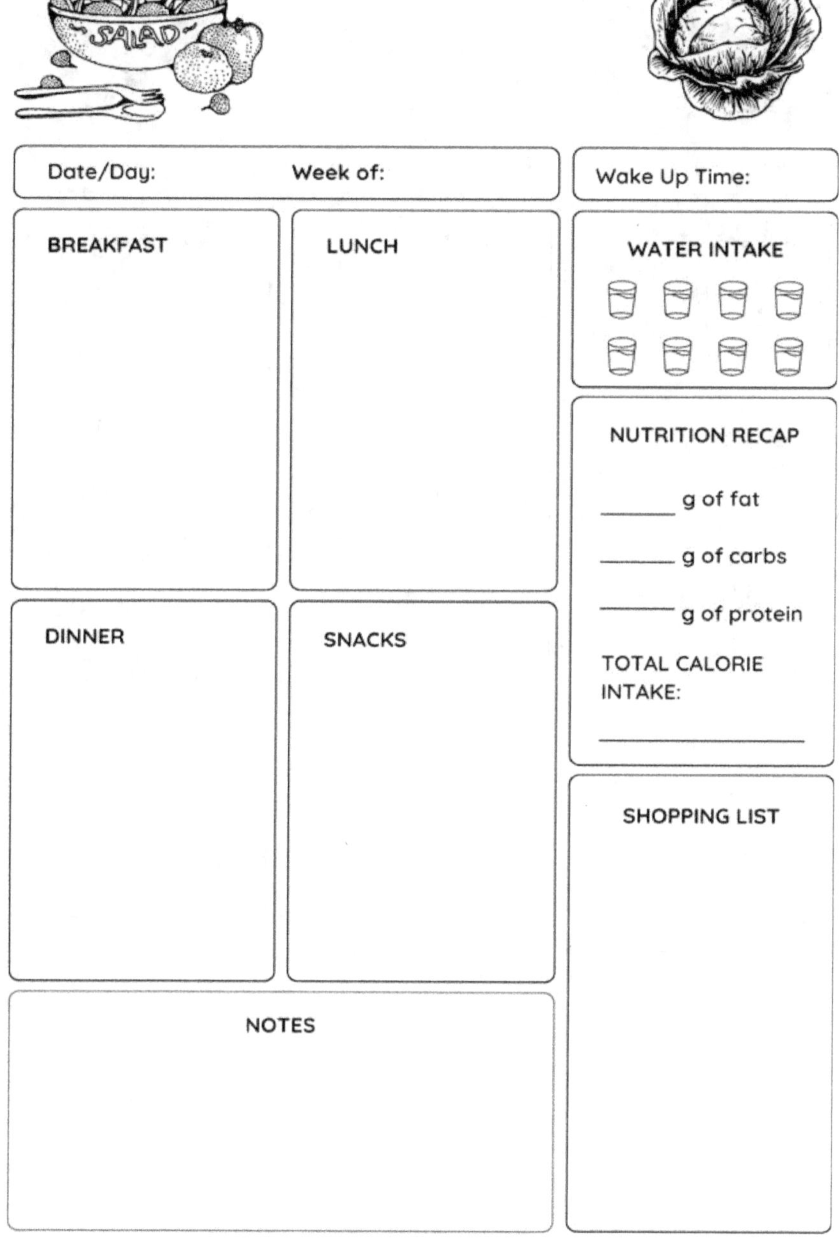

Date/Day:	Week of:

Wake Up Time:

BREAKFAST

LUNCH

WATER INTAKE

NUTRITION RECAP

_________ g of fat

_________ g of carbs

_________ g of protein

TOTAL CALORIE INTAKE:

____

DINNER

SNACKS

SHOPPING LIST

NOTES

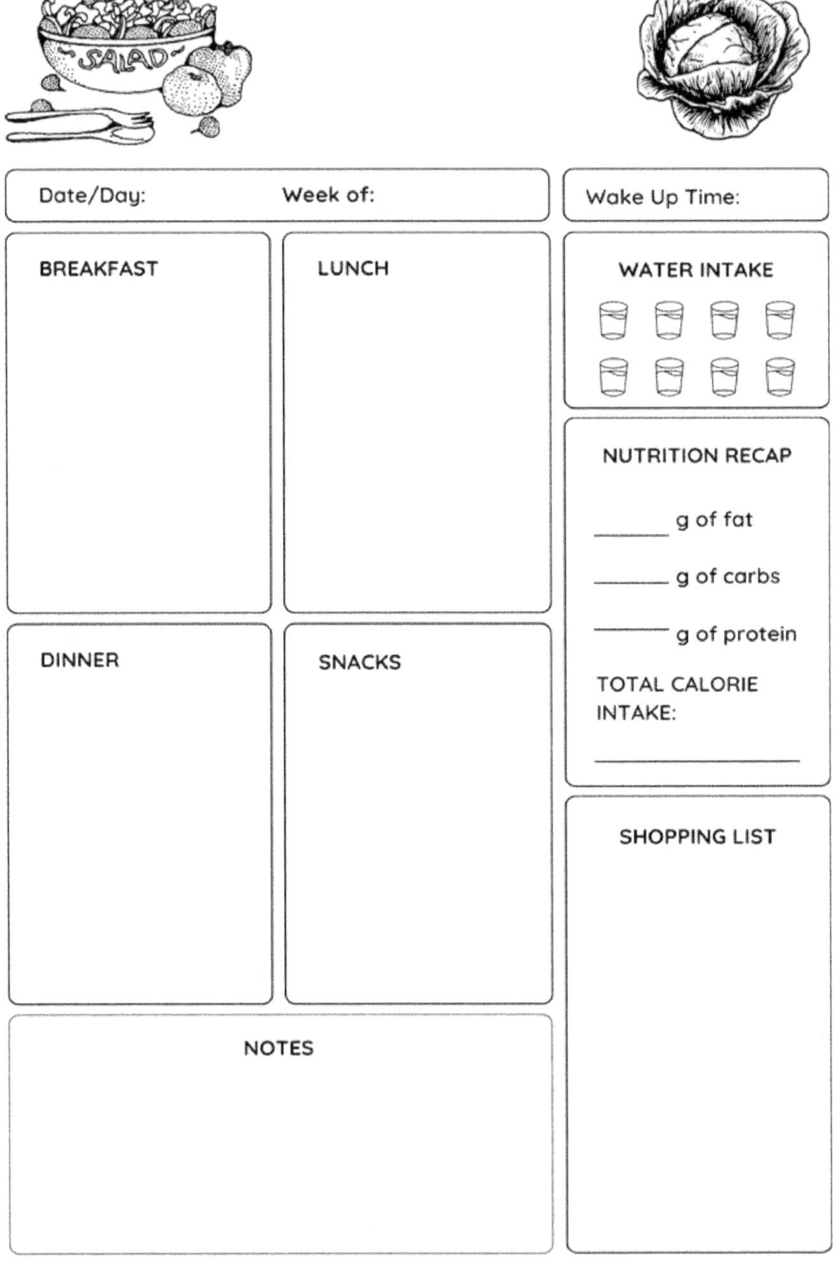

| Date/Day: | Week of: | Wake Up Time: |

BREAKFAST

LUNCH

WATER INTAKE

NUTRITION RECAP

_______ g of fat

_______ g of carbs

_______ g of protein

TOTAL CALORIE INTAKE:

DINNER

SNACKS

SHOPPING LIST

NOTES

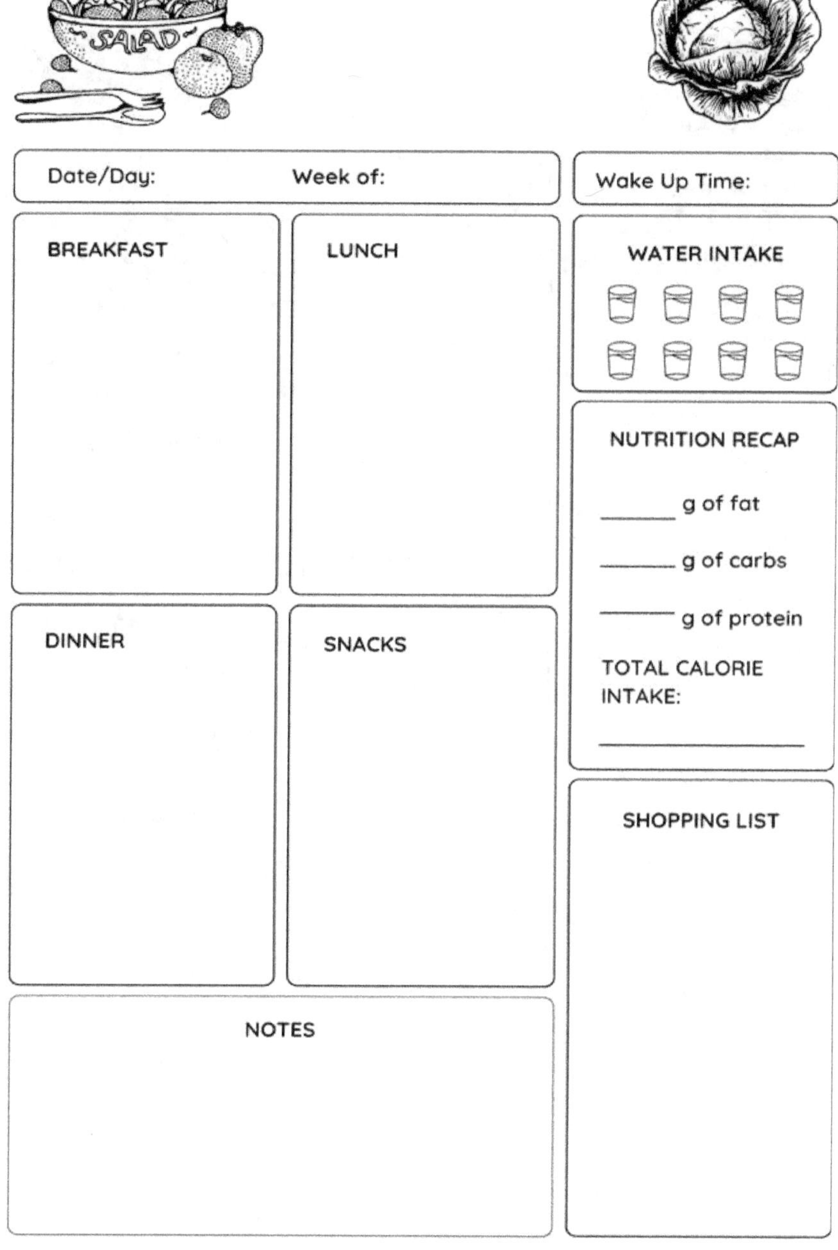

Date/Day: Week of:

Wake Up Time:

BREAKFAST

LUNCH

WATER INTAKE

NUTRITION RECAP

________ g of fat

________ g of carbs

________ g of protein

TOTAL CALORIE INTAKE:

____

DINNER

SNACKS

SHOPPING LIST

NOTES

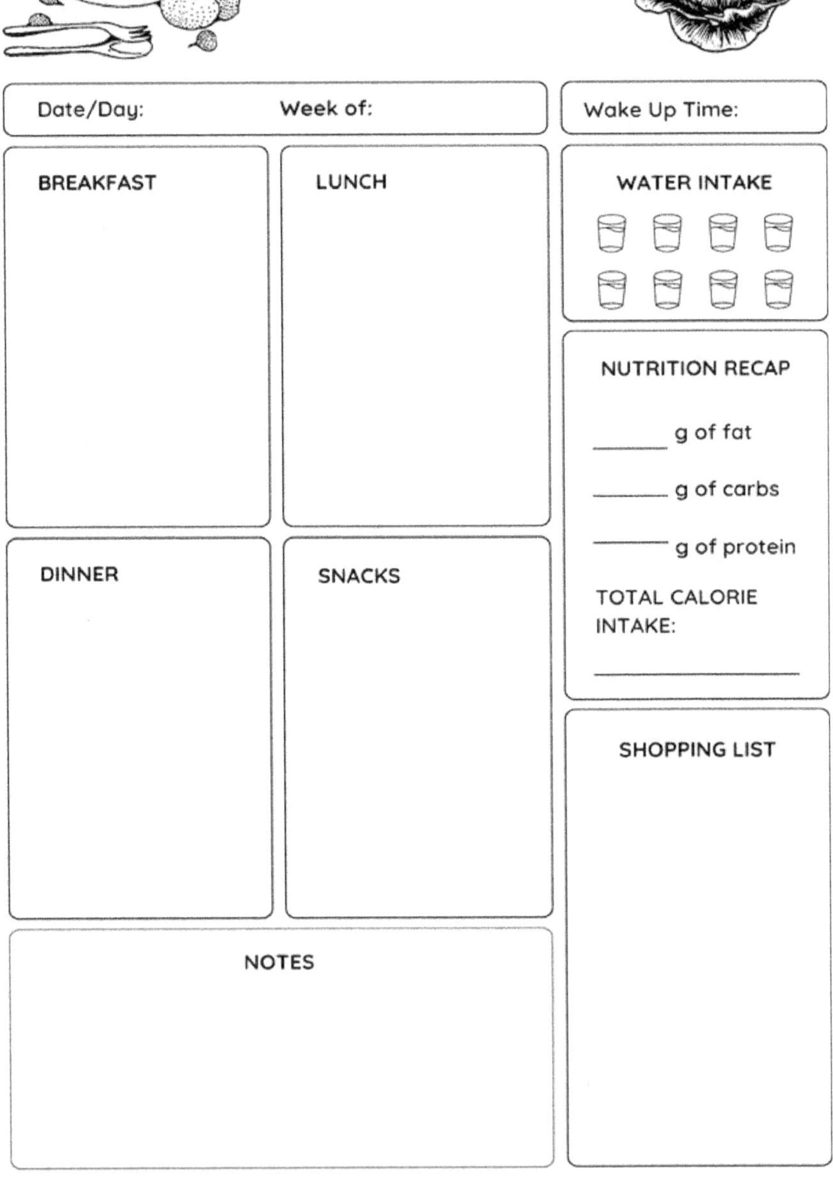

| Date/Day: | Week of: | Wake Up Time: |

BREAKFAST

LUNCH

WATER INTAKE

NUTRITION RECAP

_______ g of fat

_______ g of carbs

_______ g of protein

TOTAL CALORIE INTAKE:

____

DINNER

SNACKS

SHOPPING LIST

NOTES

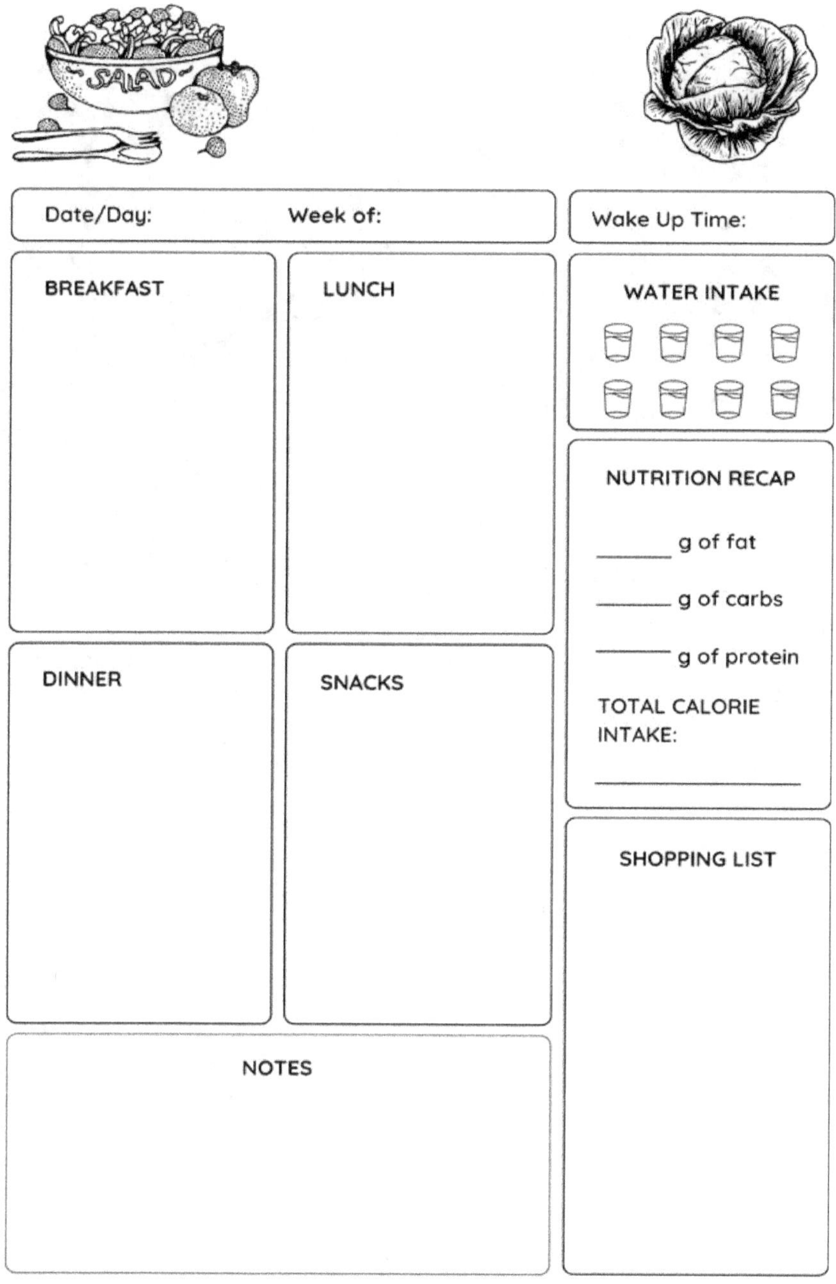

Date/Day: Week of:

Wake Up Time:

BREAKFAST

LUNCH

WATER INTAKE

NUTRITION RECAP

_______ g of fat

_______ g of carbs

_______ g of protein

TOTAL CALORIE INTAKE:

____

DINNER

SNACKS

SHOPPING LIST

NOTES

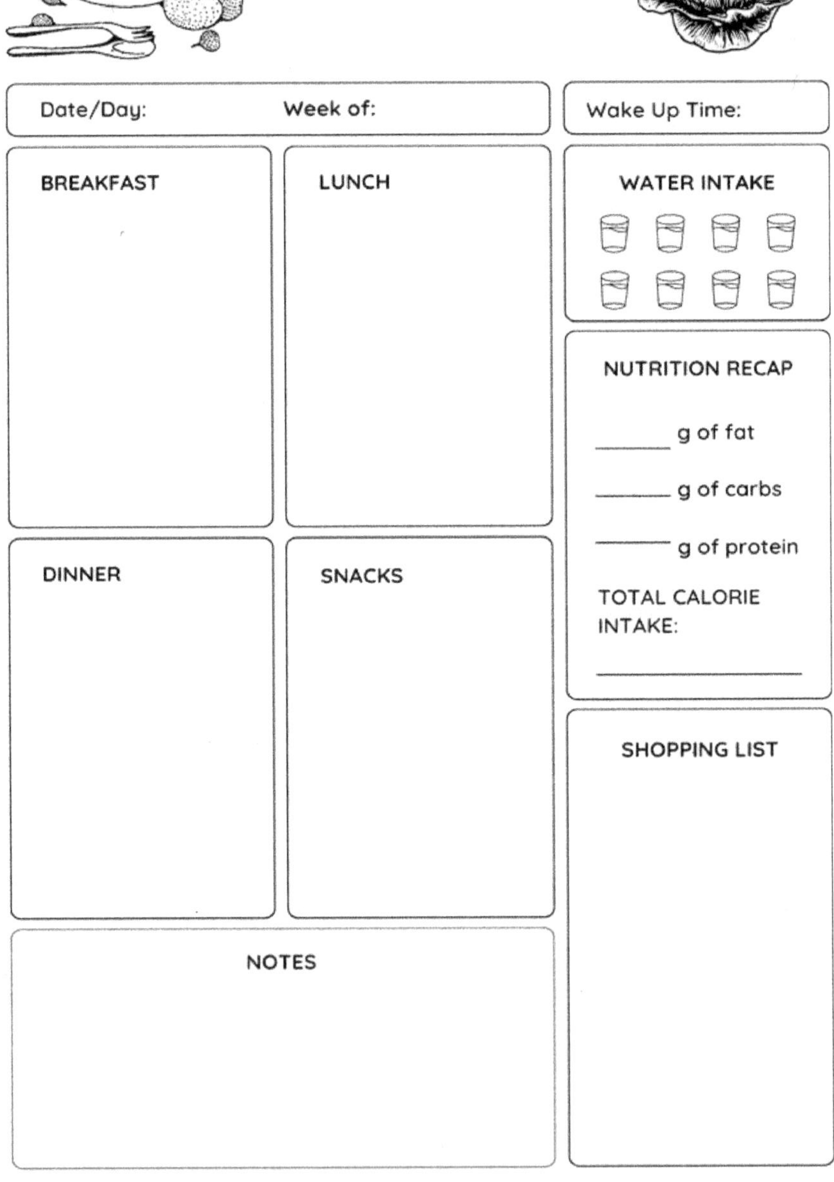

| Date/Day: | Week of: | Wake Up Time: |

BREAKFAST

LUNCH

WATER INTAKE

NUTRITION RECAP

__________ g of fat

__________ g of carbs

__________ g of protein

TOTAL CALORIE INTAKE:

____

DINNER

SNACKS

SHOPPING LIST

NOTES

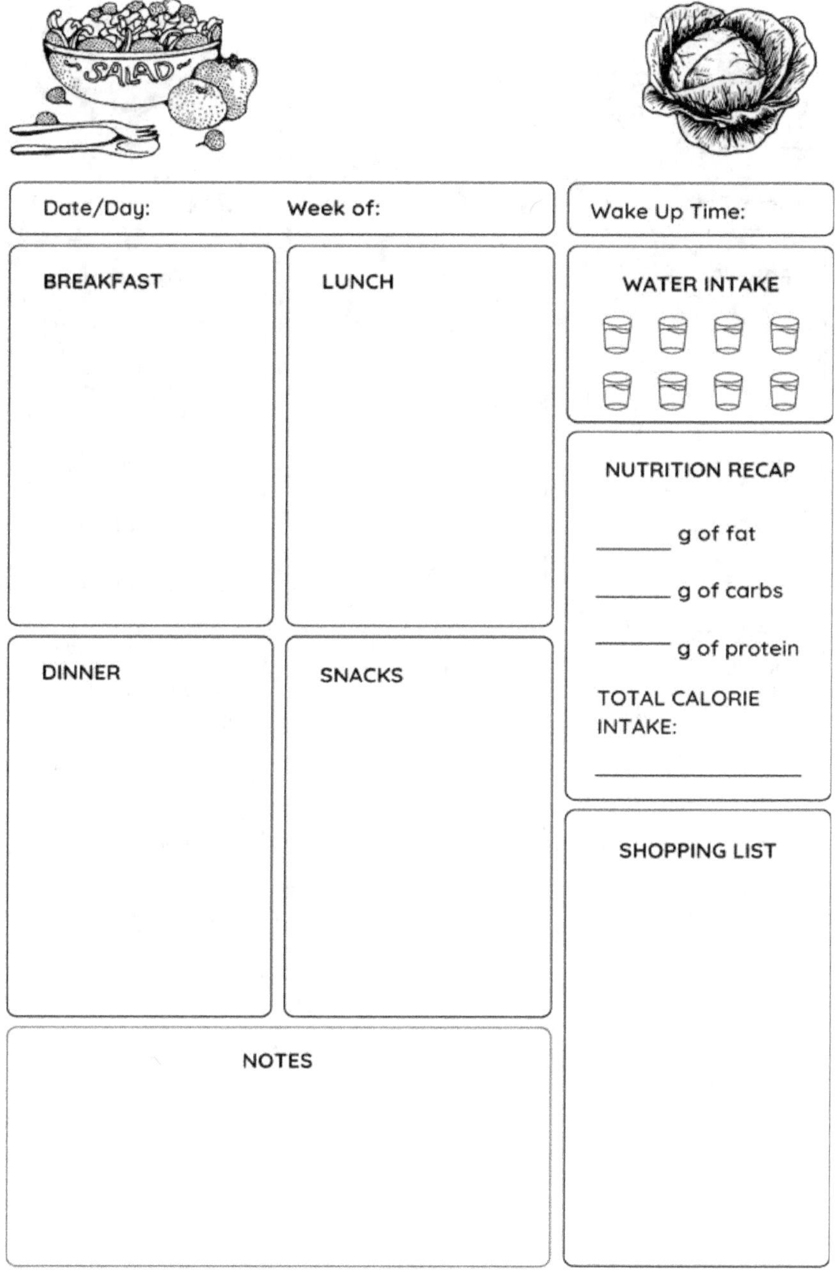

| Date/Day: | Week of: | Wake Up Time: |

BREAKFAST

LUNCH

WATER INTAKE

NUTRITION RECAP

_______ g of fat

_______ g of carbs

_______ g of protein

TOTAL CALORIE INTAKE:

____

DINNER

SNACKS

SHOPPING LIST

NOTES

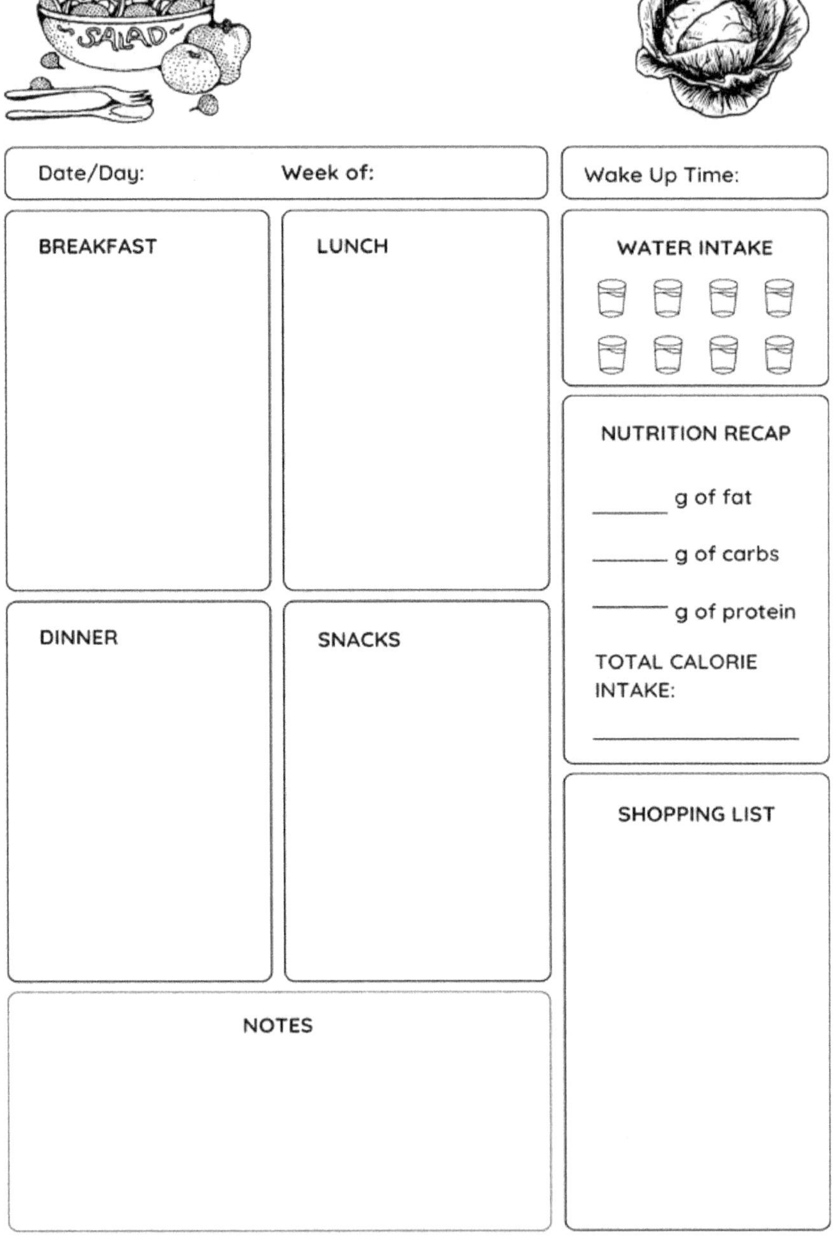

| Date/Day: | Week of: | Wake Up Time: |

BREAKFAST

LUNCH

WATER INTAKE

NUTRITION RECAP

_______ g of fat

_______ g of carbs

_______ g of protein

TOTAL CALORIE INTAKE:

____

DINNER

SNACKS

SHOPPING LIST

NOTES

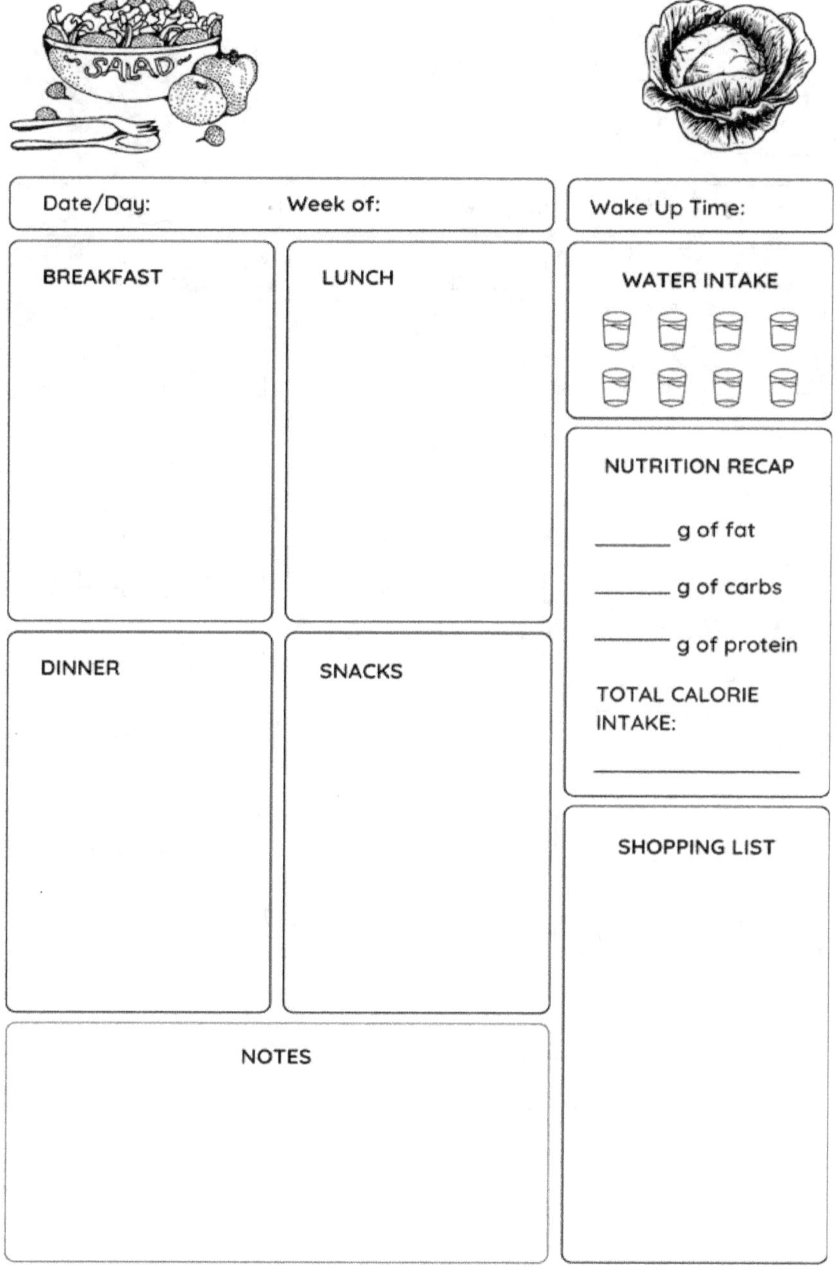

Date/Day:
Week of:
Wake Up Time:
BREAKFAST
LUNCH
WATER INTAKE
NUTRITION RECAP
_______ g of fat
_______ g of carbs
_______ g of protein
TOTAL CALORIE INTAKE:
DINNER
SNACKS
SHOPPING LIST
NOTES

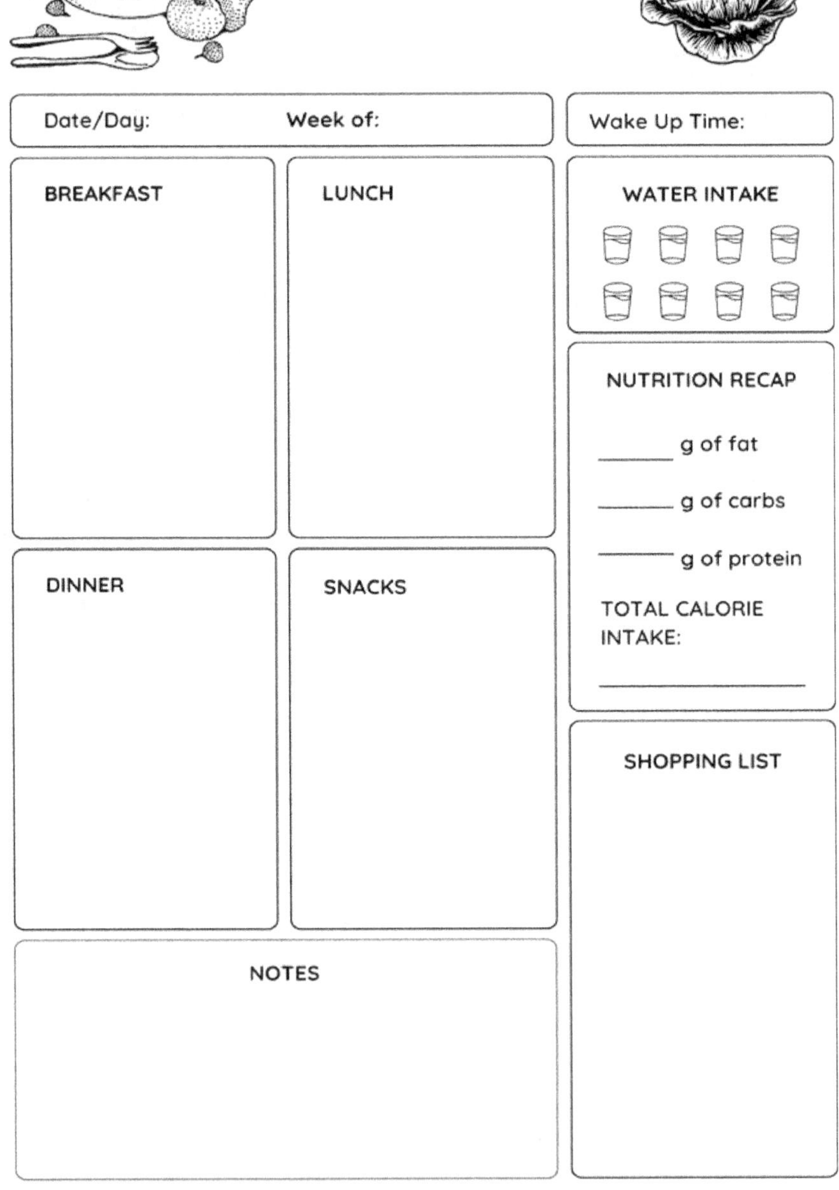

| Date/Day: | Week of: | Wake Up Time: |

BREAKFAST

LUNCH

WATER INTAKE

NUTRITION RECAP

_______ g of fat

_______ g of carbs

_______ g of protein

TOTAL CALORIE INTAKE:

____

DINNER

SNACKS

SHOPPING LIST

NOTES

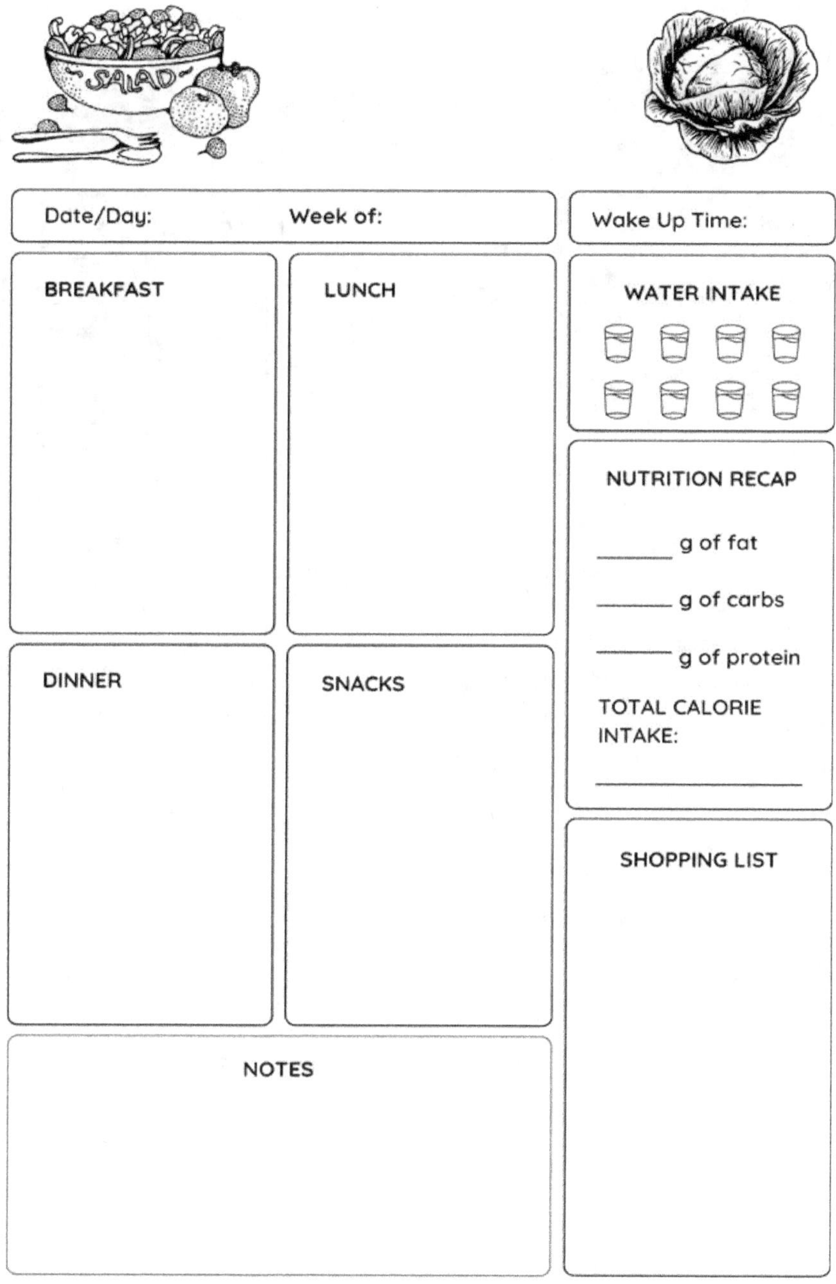

| Date/Day: | Week of: | Wake Up Time: |

BREAKFAST

LUNCH

WATER INTAKE

NUTRITION RECAP

__________ g of fat

__________ g of carbs

__________ g of protein

TOTAL CALORIE INTAKE:

____

DINNER

SNACKS

SHOPPING LIST

NOTES

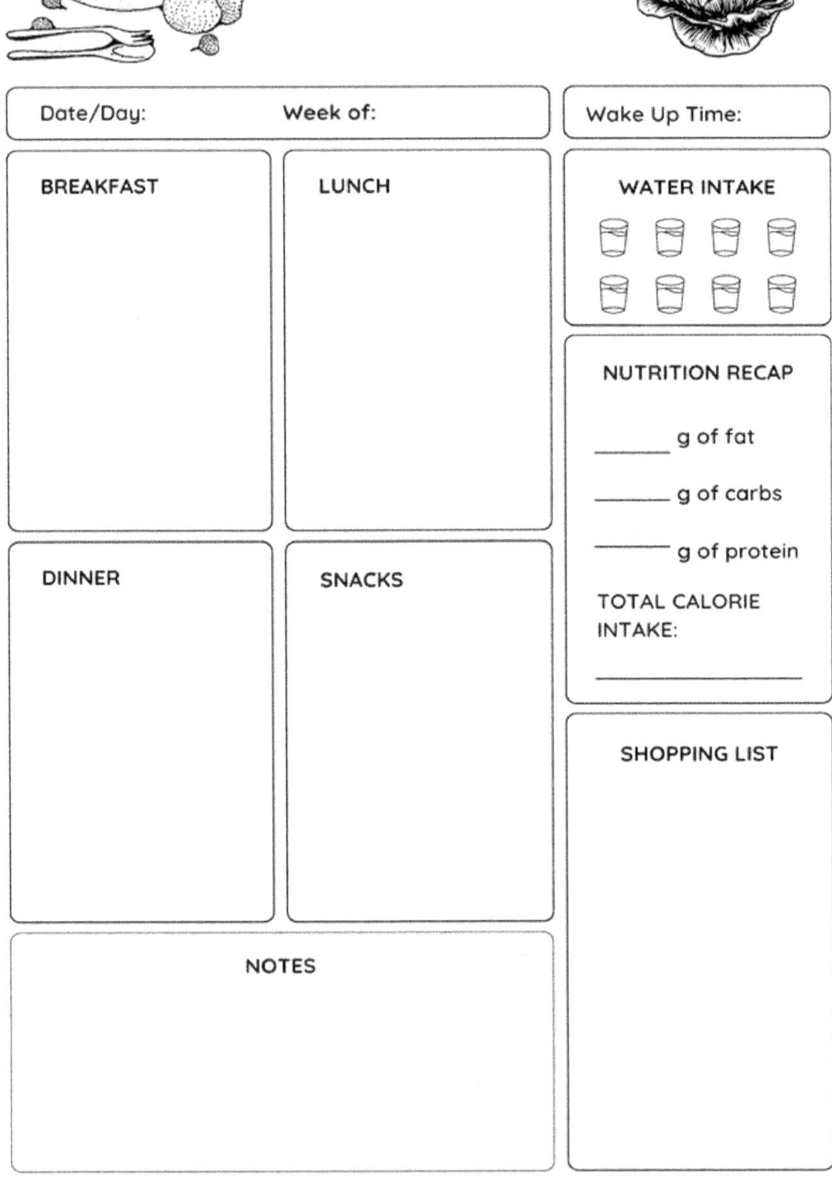

| Date/Day: | Week of: | Wake Up Time: |

BREAKFAST

LUNCH

WATER INTAKE

NUTRITION RECAP

_________ g of fat

_________ g of carbs

_________ g of protein

TOTAL CALORIE INTAKE:

____

DINNER

SNACKS

SHOPPING LIST

NOTES

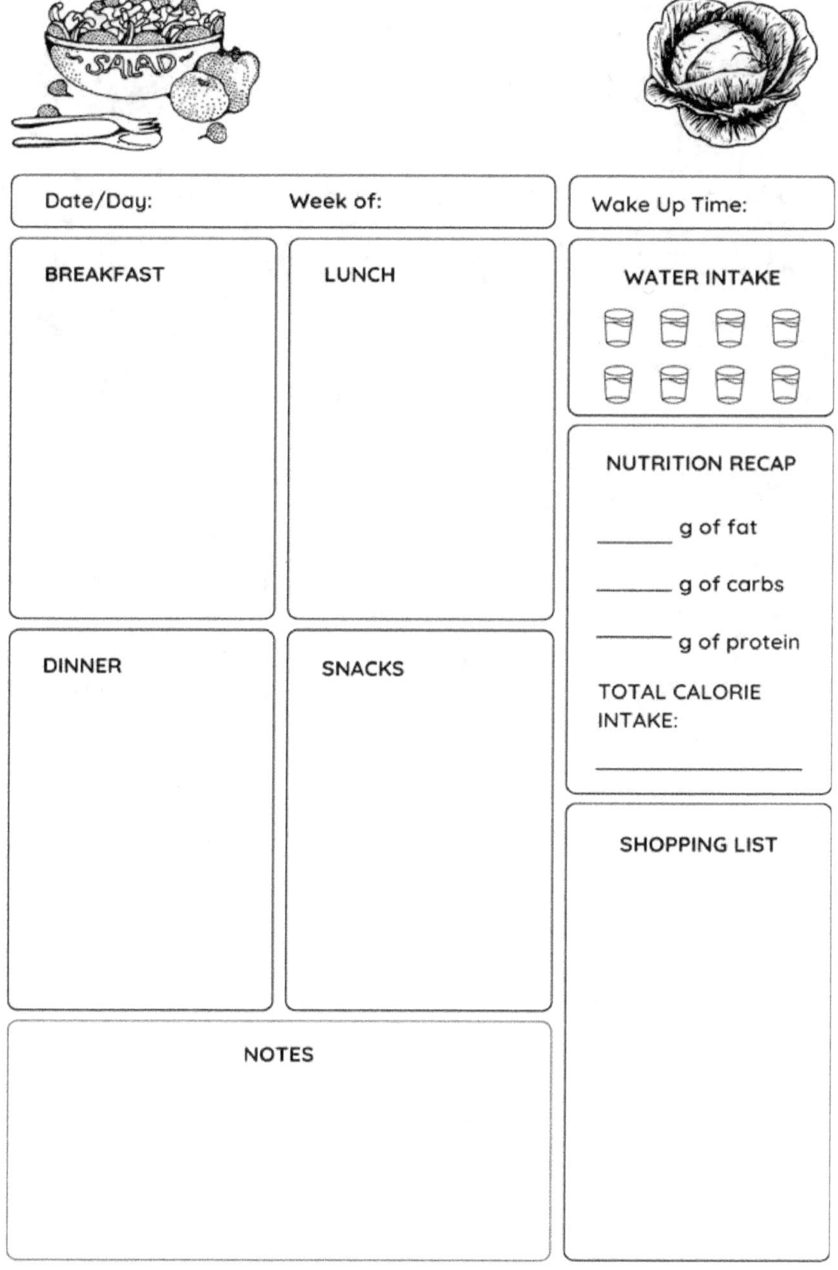

Date/Day:	Week of:

Wake Up Time:

BREAKFAST

LUNCH

DINNER

SNACKS

NOTES

WATER INTAKE

NUTRITION RECAP

_______ g of fat

_______ g of carbs

_______ g of protein

TOTAL CALORIE INTAKE:

____

SHOPPING LIST

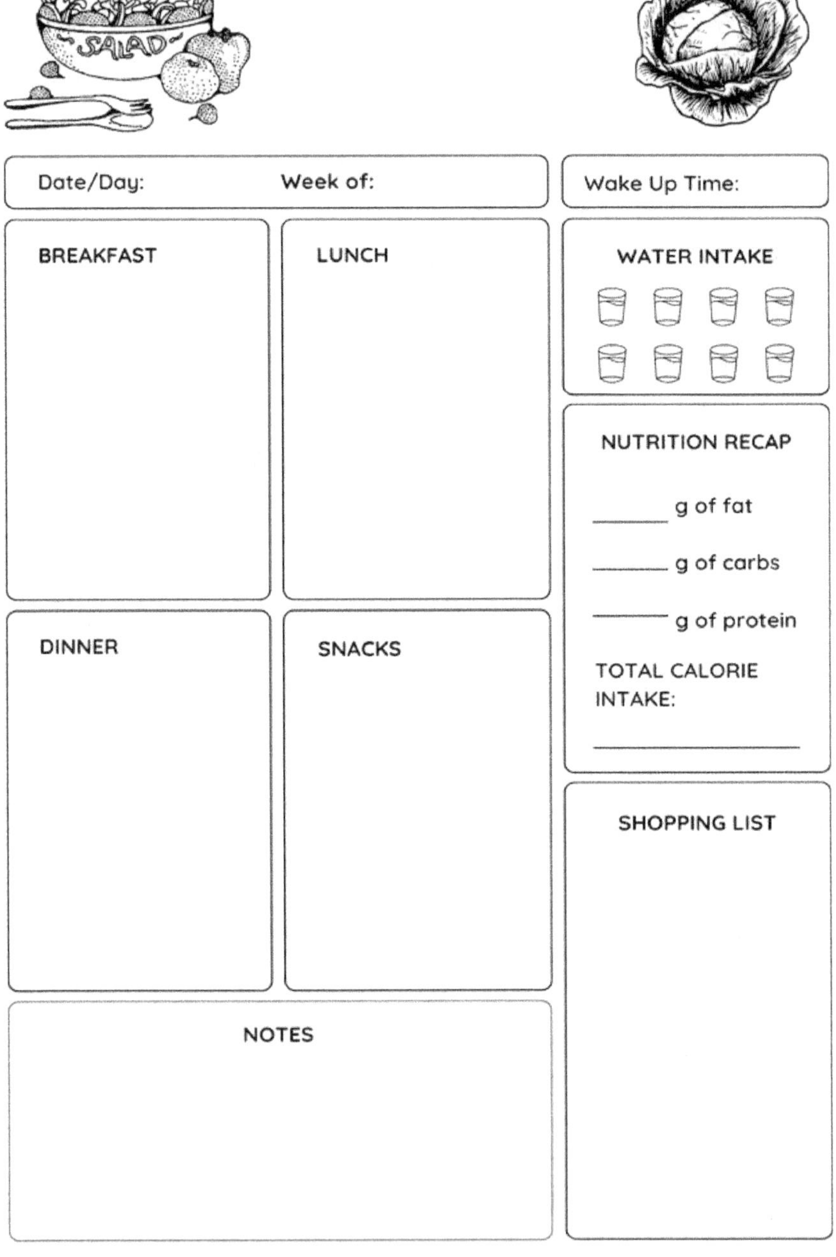

Date/Day:
Week of:
Wake Up Time:
BREAKFAST
LUNCH
WATER INTAKE
NUTRITION RECAP
_______ g of fat
_______ g of carbs
_______ g of protein
TOTAL CALORIE INTAKE:
DINNER
SNACKS
SHOPPING LIST
NOTES

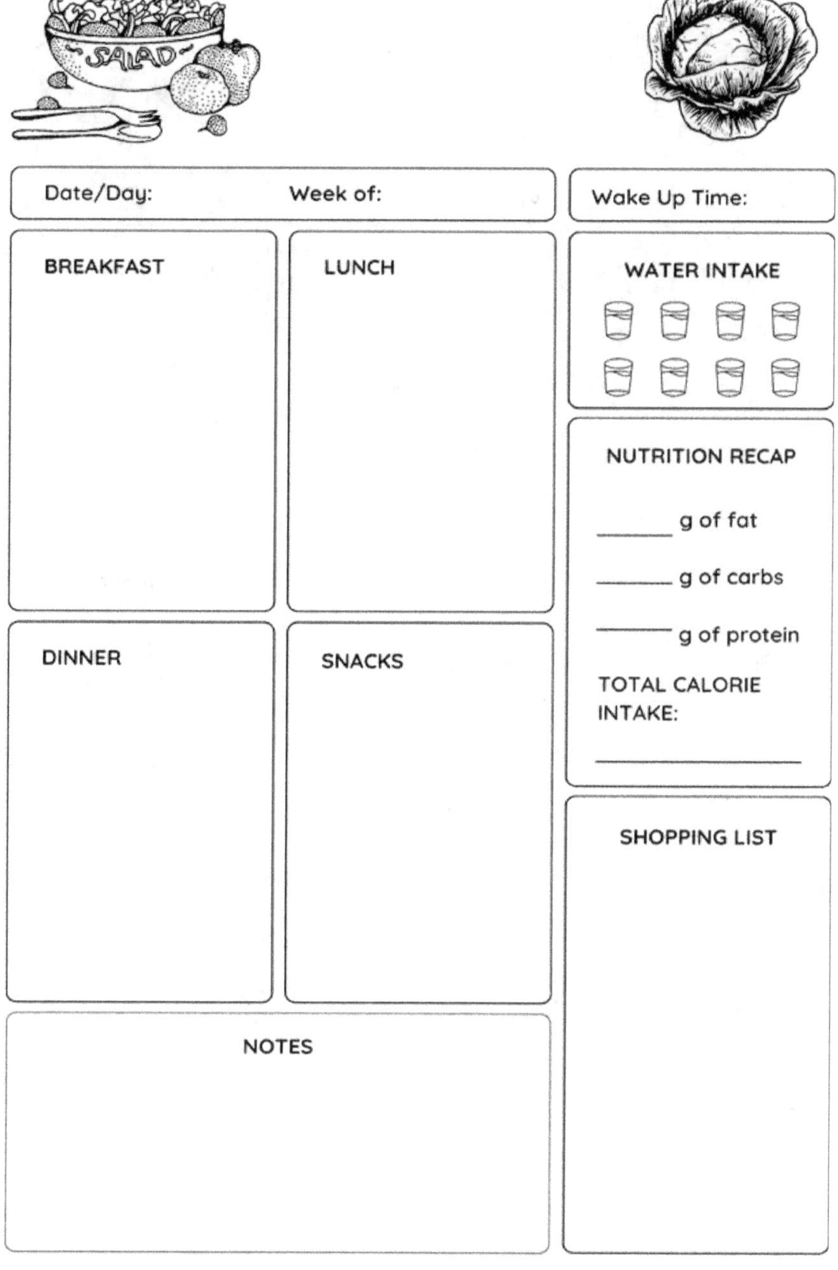
Date/Day:
Week of:
Wake Up Time:
BREAKFAST
LUNCH
WATER INTAKE
NUTRITION RECAP
_______ g of fat
_______ g of carbs
_______ g of protein
TOTAL CALORIE
INTAKE:
DINNER
SNACKS
SHOPPING LIST
NOTES

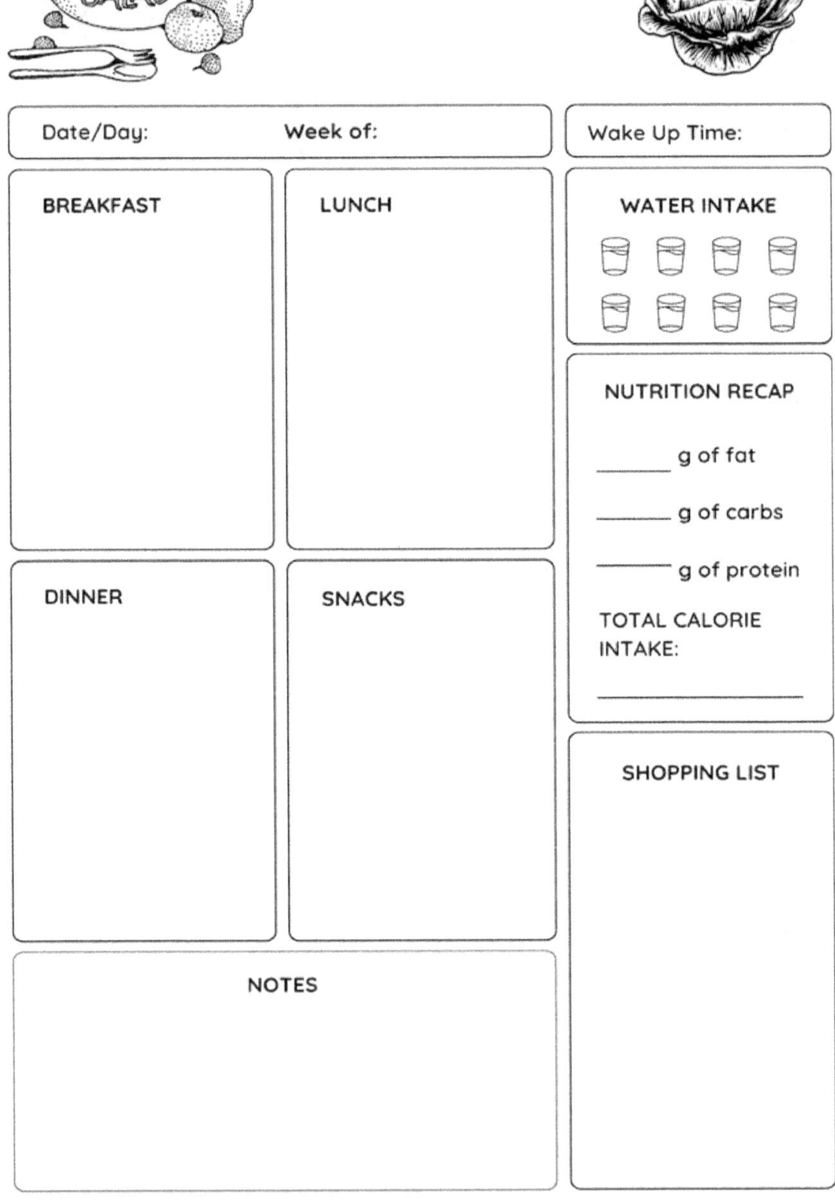

| Date/Day: | Week of: | Wake Up Time: |

BREAKFAST

LUNCH

WATER INTAKE

NUTRITION RECAP

_________ g of fat

_________ g of carbs

_________ g of protein

TOTAL CALORIE INTAKE:

____

DINNER

SNACKS

SHOPPING LIST

NOTES

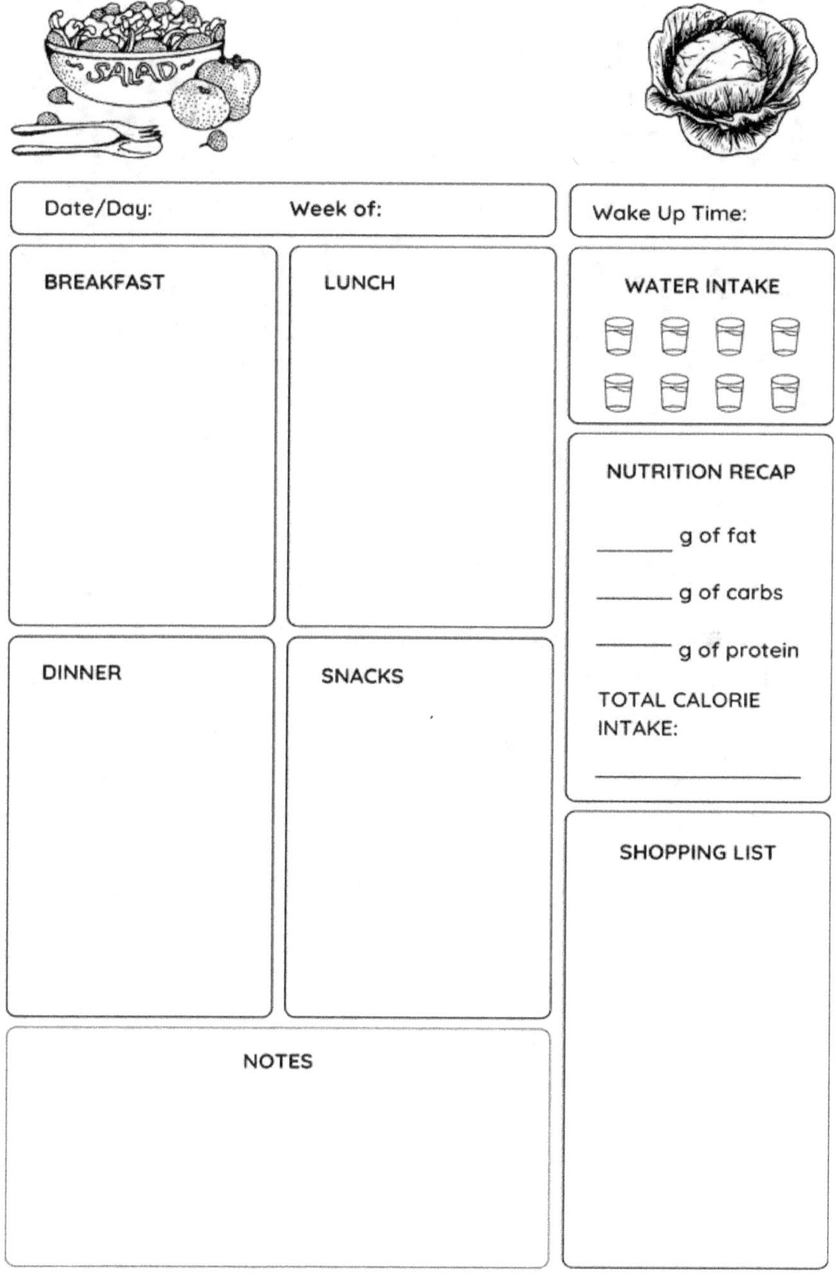

| Date/Day: | Week of: | Wake Up Time: |

BREAKFAST

LUNCH

WATER INTAKE

NUTRITION RECAP

_______ g of fat

_______ g of carbs

_______ g of protein

TOTAL CALORIE INTAKE:

____

DINNER

SNACKS

SHOPPING LIST

NOTES

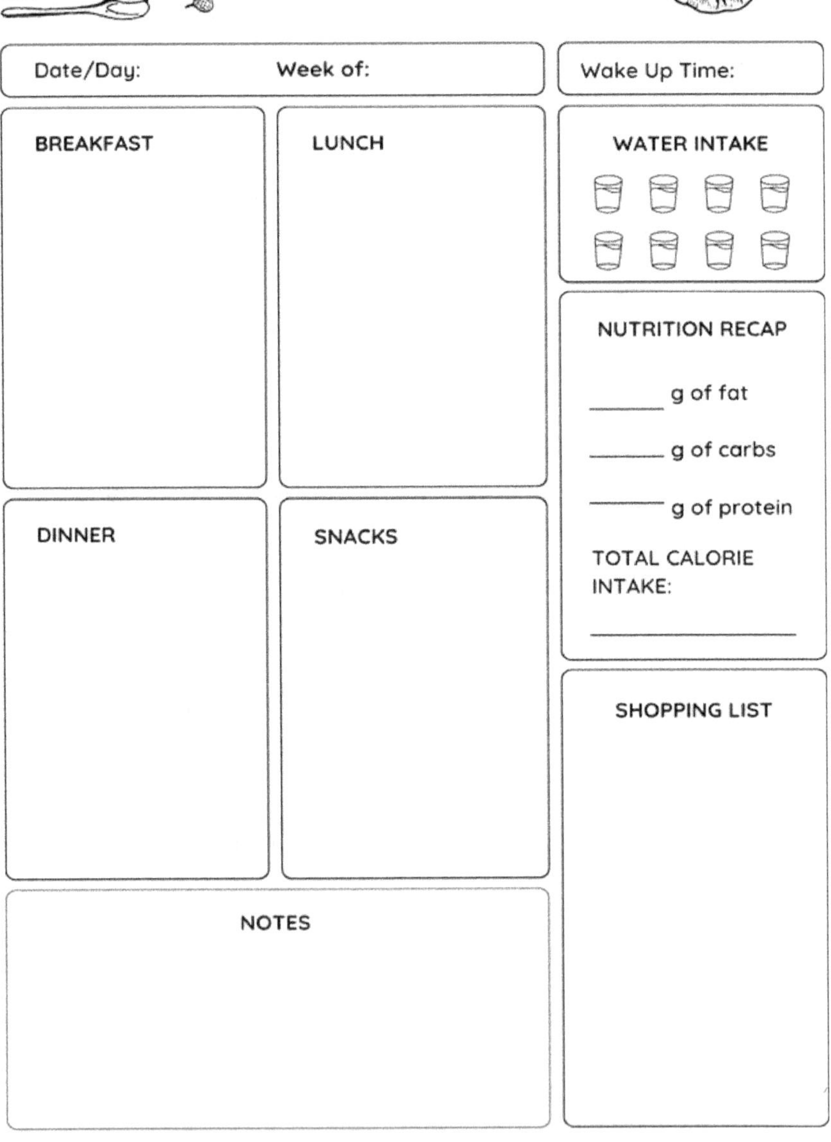

| Date/Day: | Week of: | Wake Up Time: |

BREAKFAST

LUNCH

WATER INTAKE

NUTRITION RECAP

_______ g of fat

_______ g of carbs

_______ g of protein

TOTAL CALORIE INTAKE:

____

DINNER

SNACKS

SHOPPING LIST

NOTES

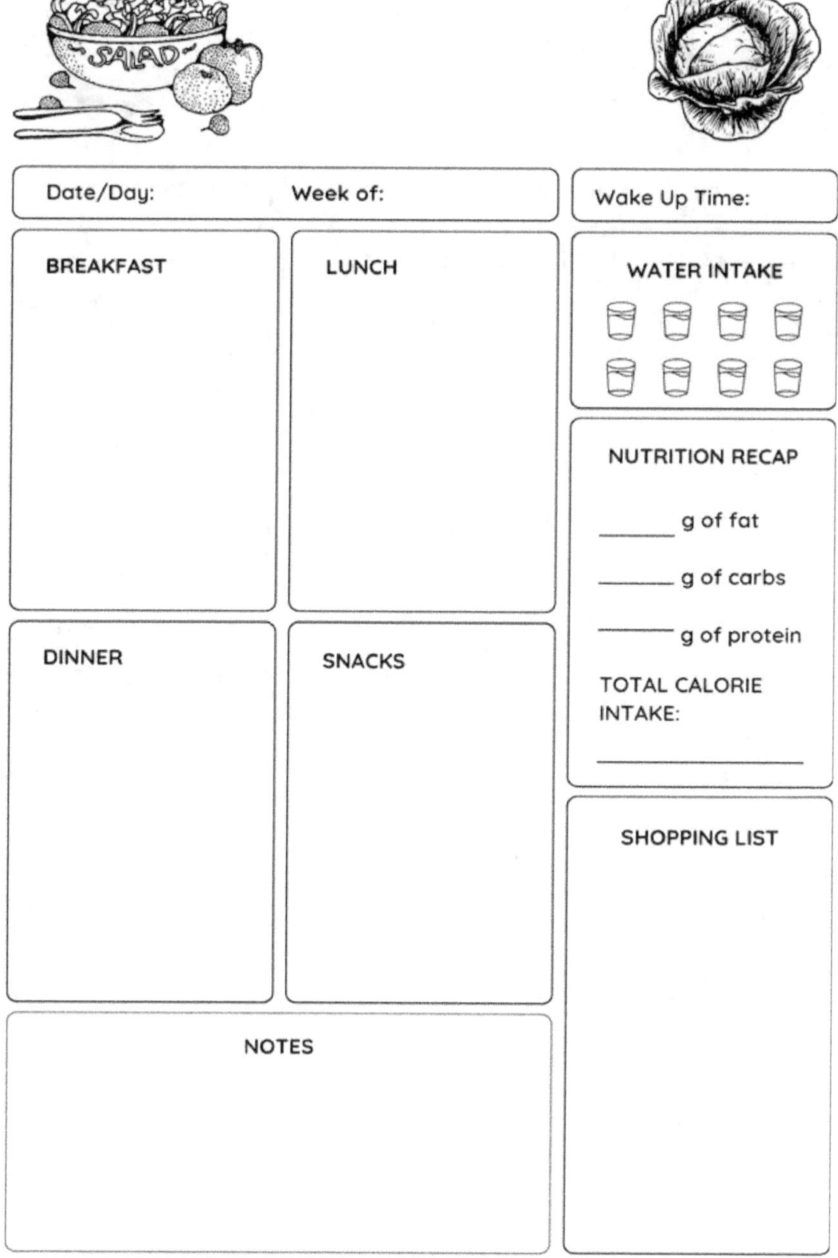

Date/Day: **Week of:**

Wake Up Time:

BREAKFAST

LUNCH

WATER INTAKE

NUTRITION RECAP

_________ g of fat

_________ g of carbs

_________ g of protein

TOTAL CALORIE INTAKE:

____

DINNER

SNACKS

SHOPPING LIST

NOTES

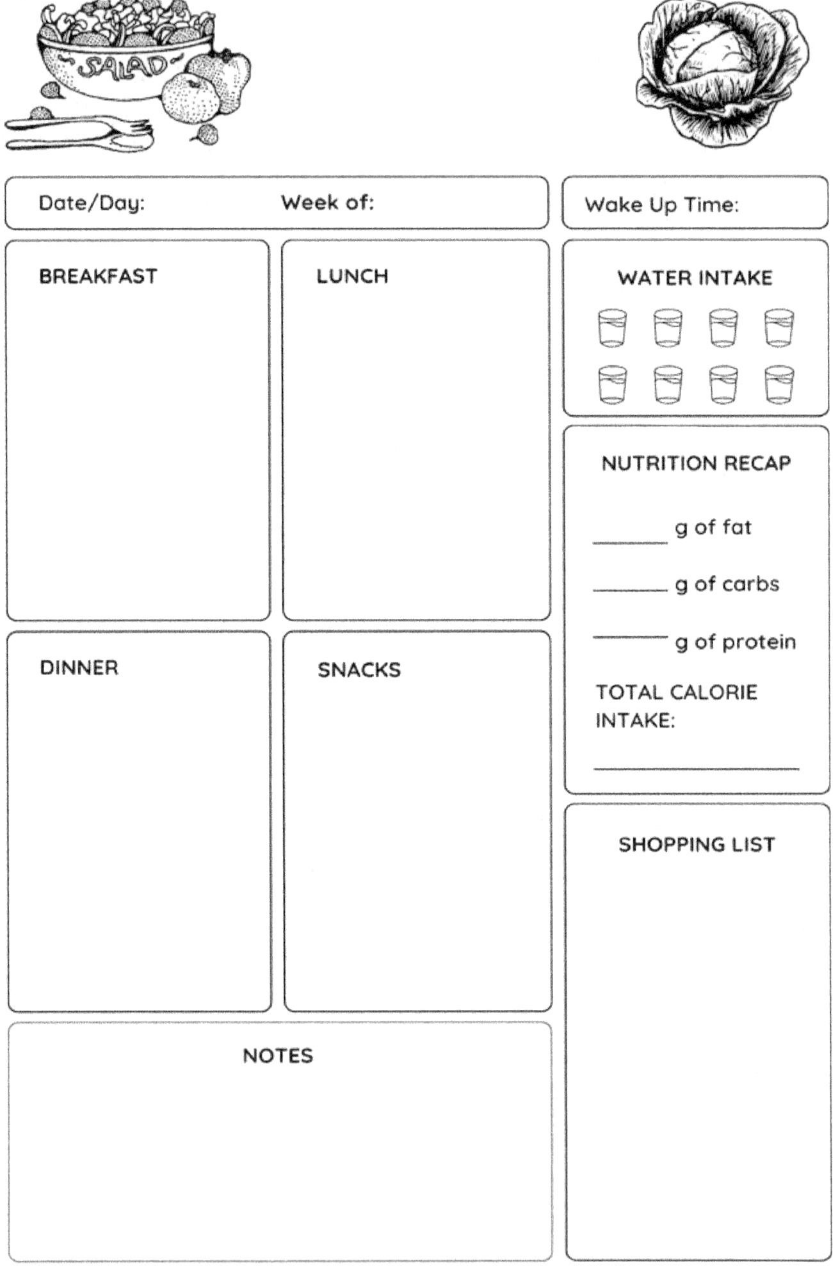

Date/Day: ___________ Week of: ___________

Wake Up Time: ___________

BREAKFAST

LUNCH

WATER INTAKE

NUTRITION RECAP

________ g of fat

________ g of carbs

________ g of protein

TOTAL CALORIE INTAKE:

____

DINNER

SNACKS

SHOPPING LIST

NOTES

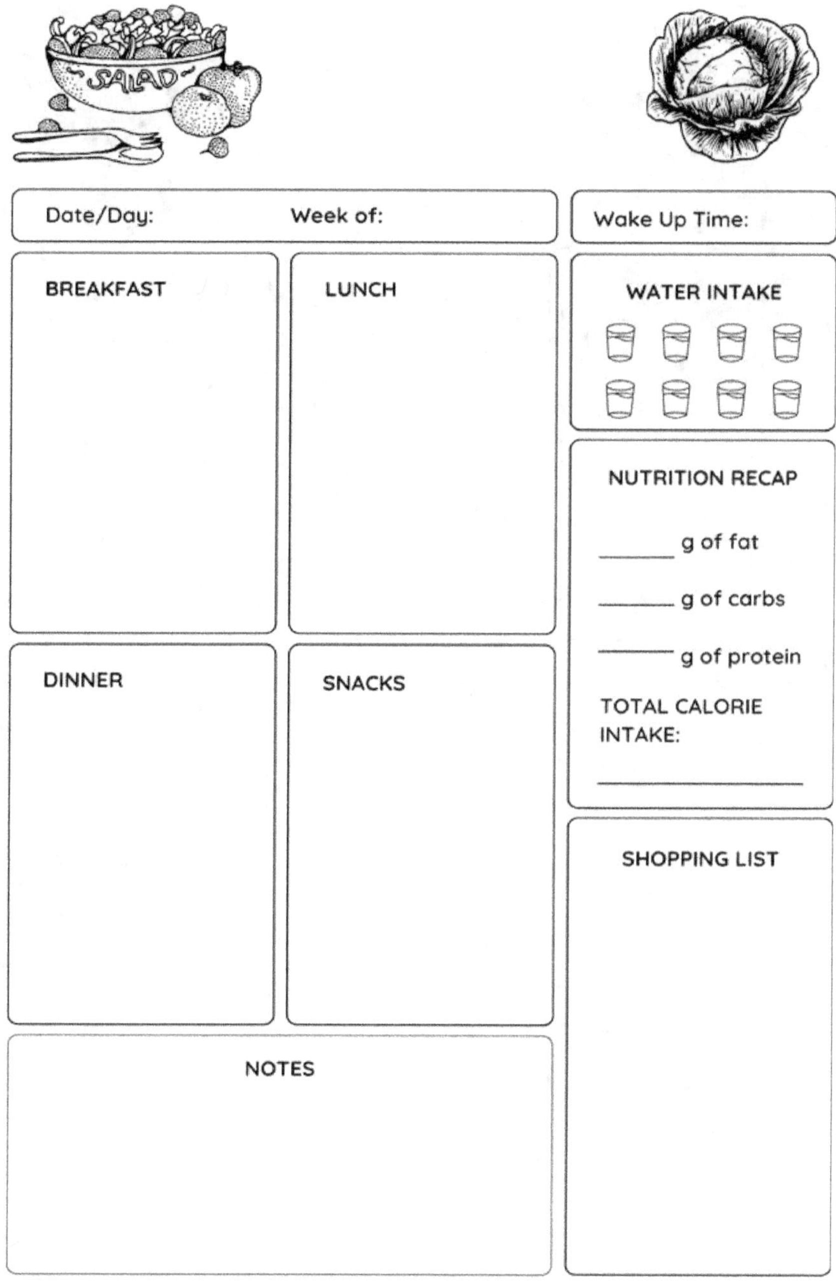

Date/Day:

Week of:

Wake Up Time:

BREAKFAST

LUNCH

WATER INTAKE

NUTRITION RECAP

_______ g of fat

_______ g of carbs

_______ g of protein

TOTAL CALORIE INTAKE:

DINNER

SNACKS

SHOPPING LIST

NOTES

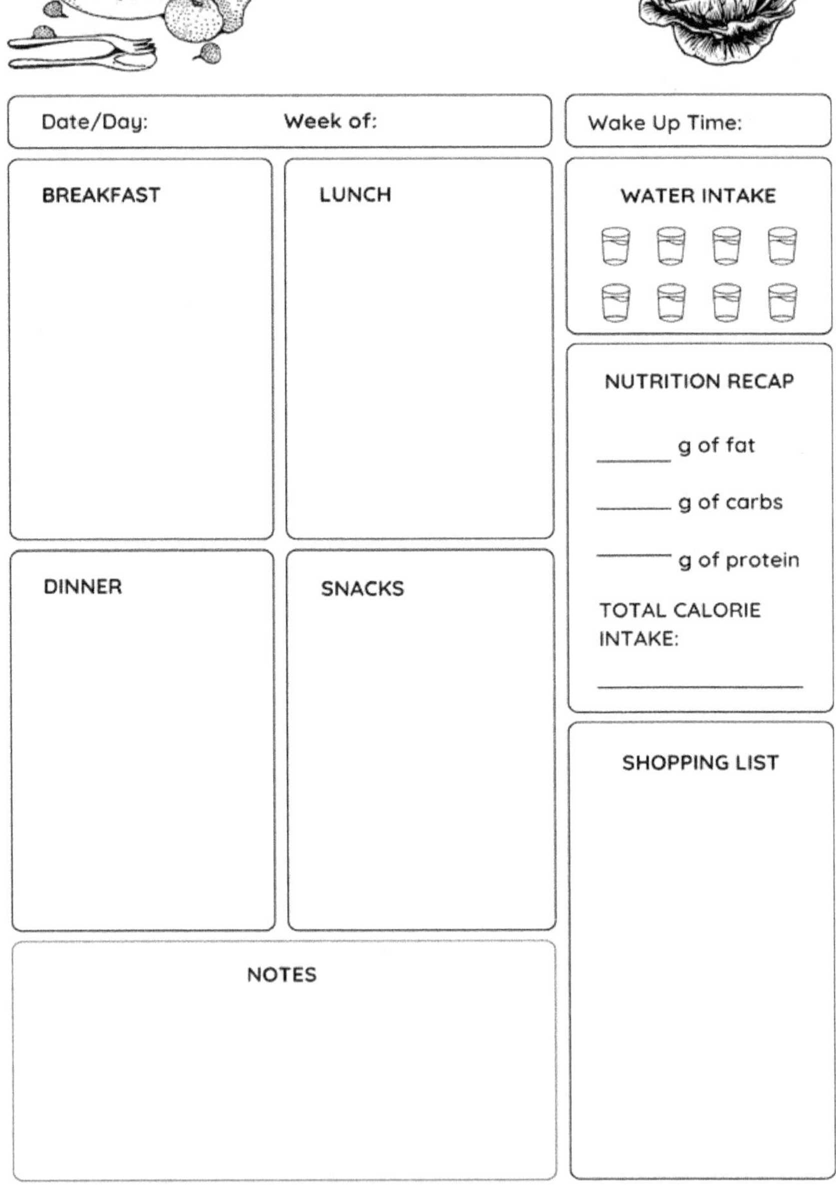

| Date/Day: | Week of: | Wake Up Time: |

BREAKFAST

LUNCH

WATER INTAKE

NUTRITION RECAP

_______ g of fat

_______ g of carbs

_______ g of protein

TOTAL CALORIE INTAKE:

____

DINNER

SNACKS

SHOPPING LIST

NOTES

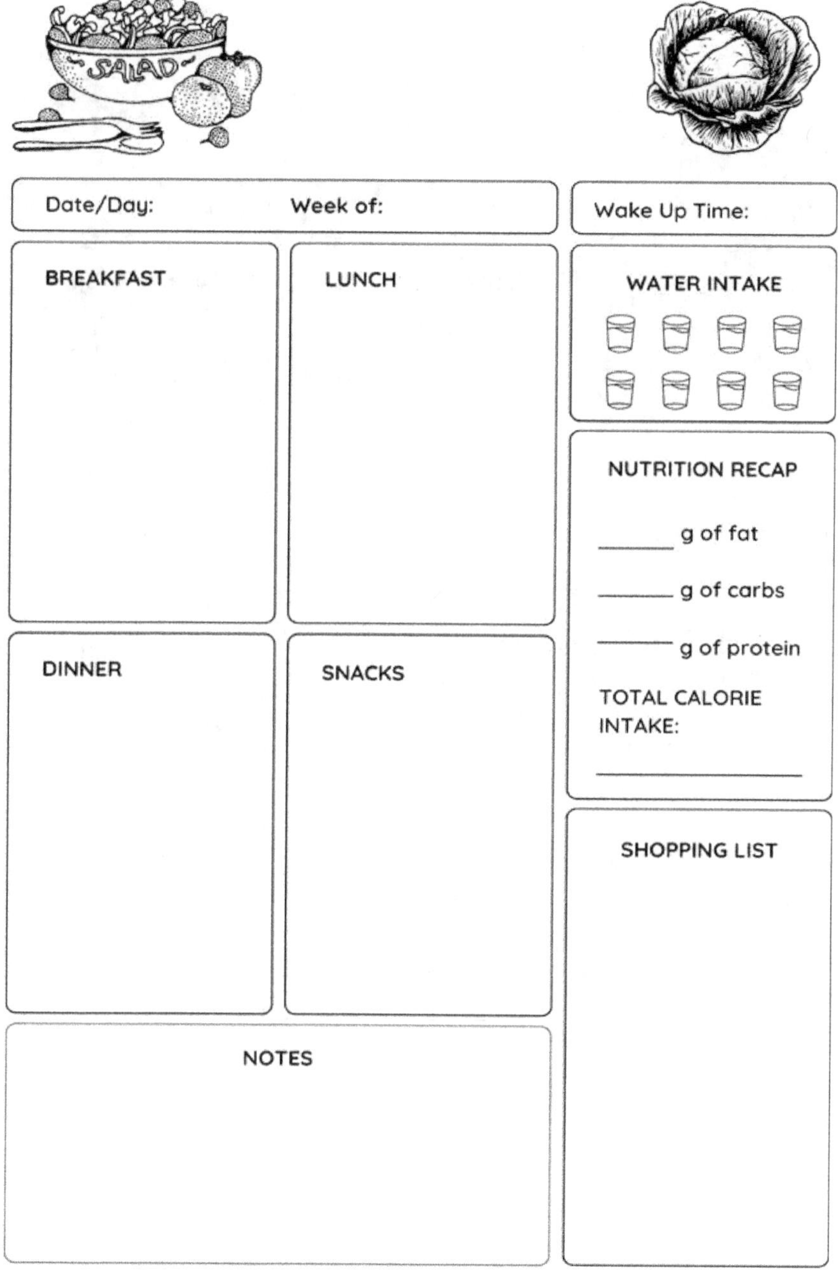

Date/Day:
Week of:
Wake Up Time:
BREAKFAST
LUNCH
WATER INTAKE
NUTRITION RECAP
________ g of fat
________ g of carbs
________ g of protein
TOTAL CALORIE INTAKE:
____
DINNER
SNACKS
SHOPPING LIST
NOTES

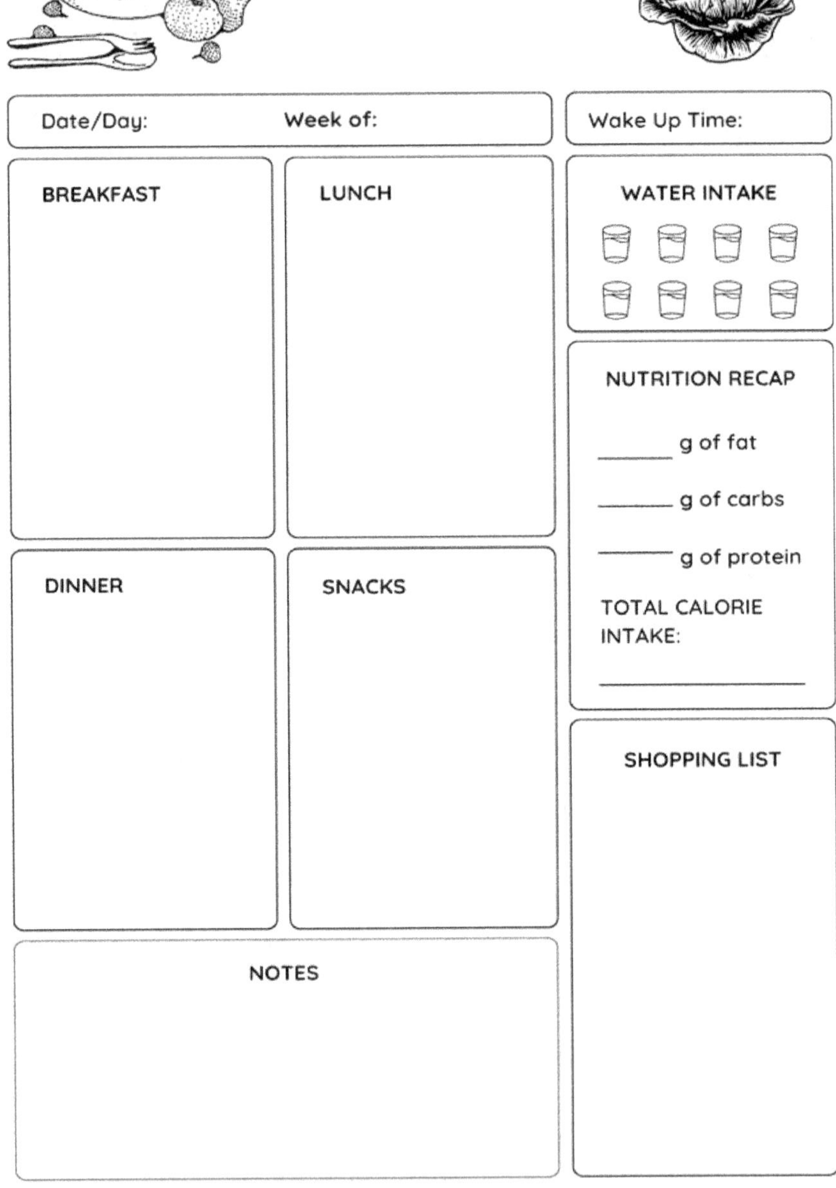

| Date/Day: | Week of: | Wake Up Time: |

BREAKFAST

LUNCH

WATER INTAKE

NUTRITION RECAP

________ g of fat

________ g of carbs

________ g of protein

TOTAL CALORIE INTAKE:

____

DINNER

SNACKS

SHOPPING LIST

NOTES

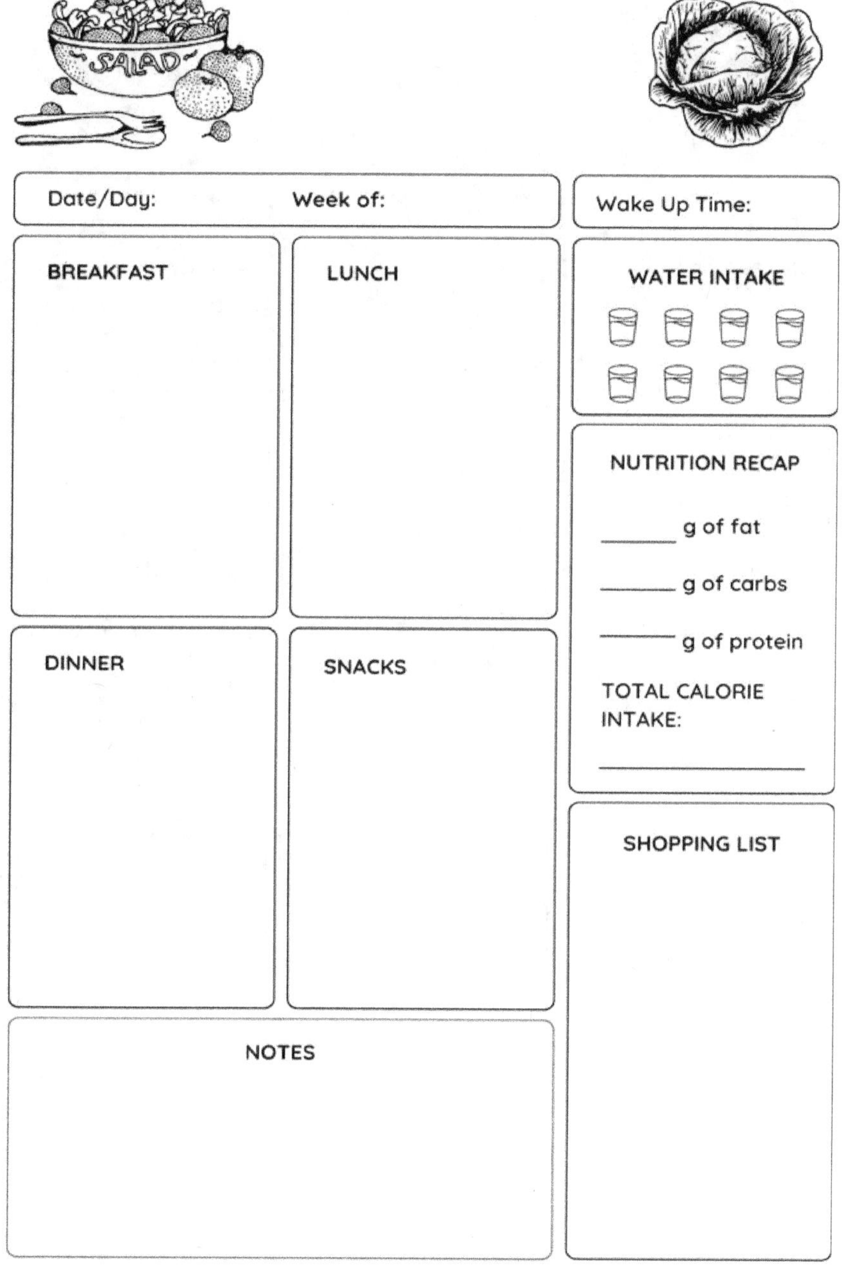

| Date/Day: | Week of: | Wake Up Time: |

BREAKFAST

LUNCH

WATER INTAKE

NUTRITION RECAP

_______ g of fat

_______ g of carbs

_______ g of protein

TOTAL CALORIE INTAKE:

____

DINNER

SNACKS

SHOPPING LIST

NOTES

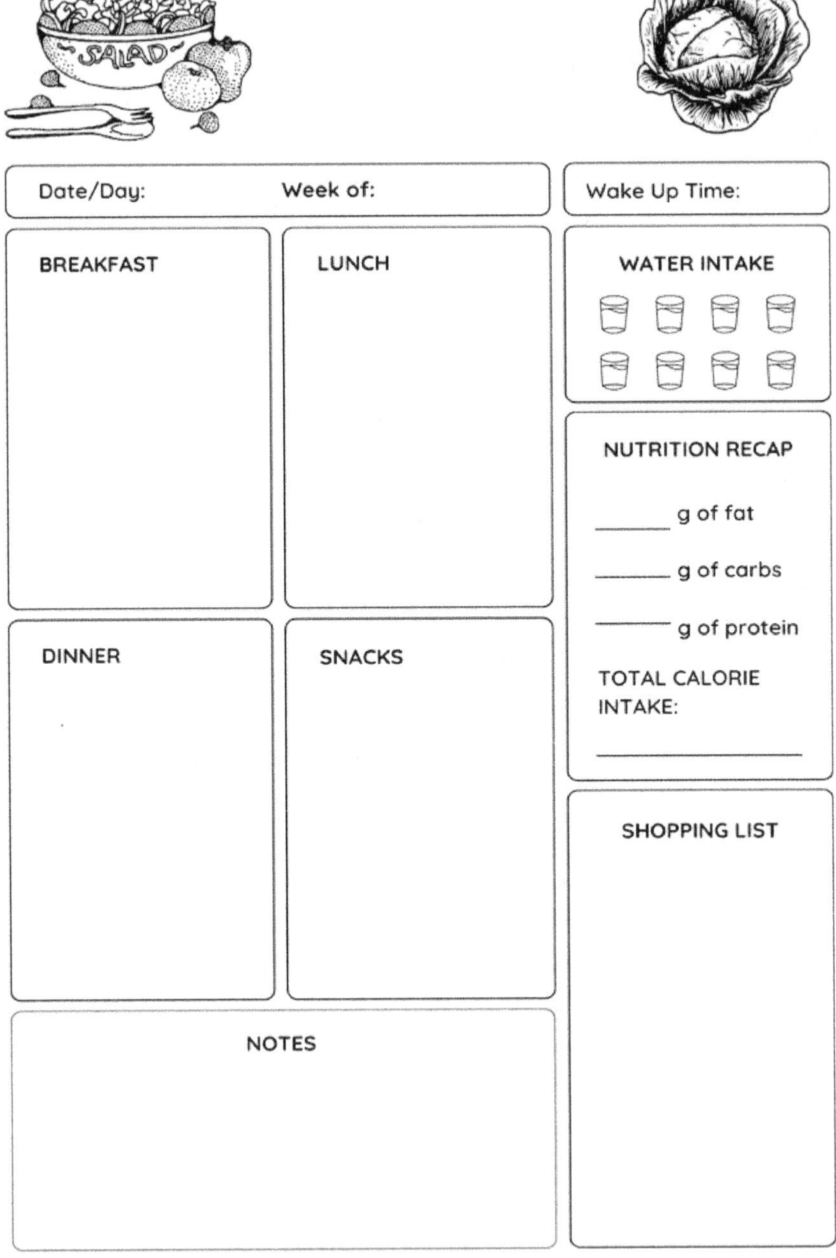

Date/Day:
Week of:
Wake Up Time:

BREAKFAST

LUNCH

WATER INTAKE

NUTRITION RECAP

_______ g of fat

_______ g of carbs

_______ g of protein

TOTAL CALORIE INTAKE:

____

DINNER

SNACKS

SHOPPING LIST

NOTES

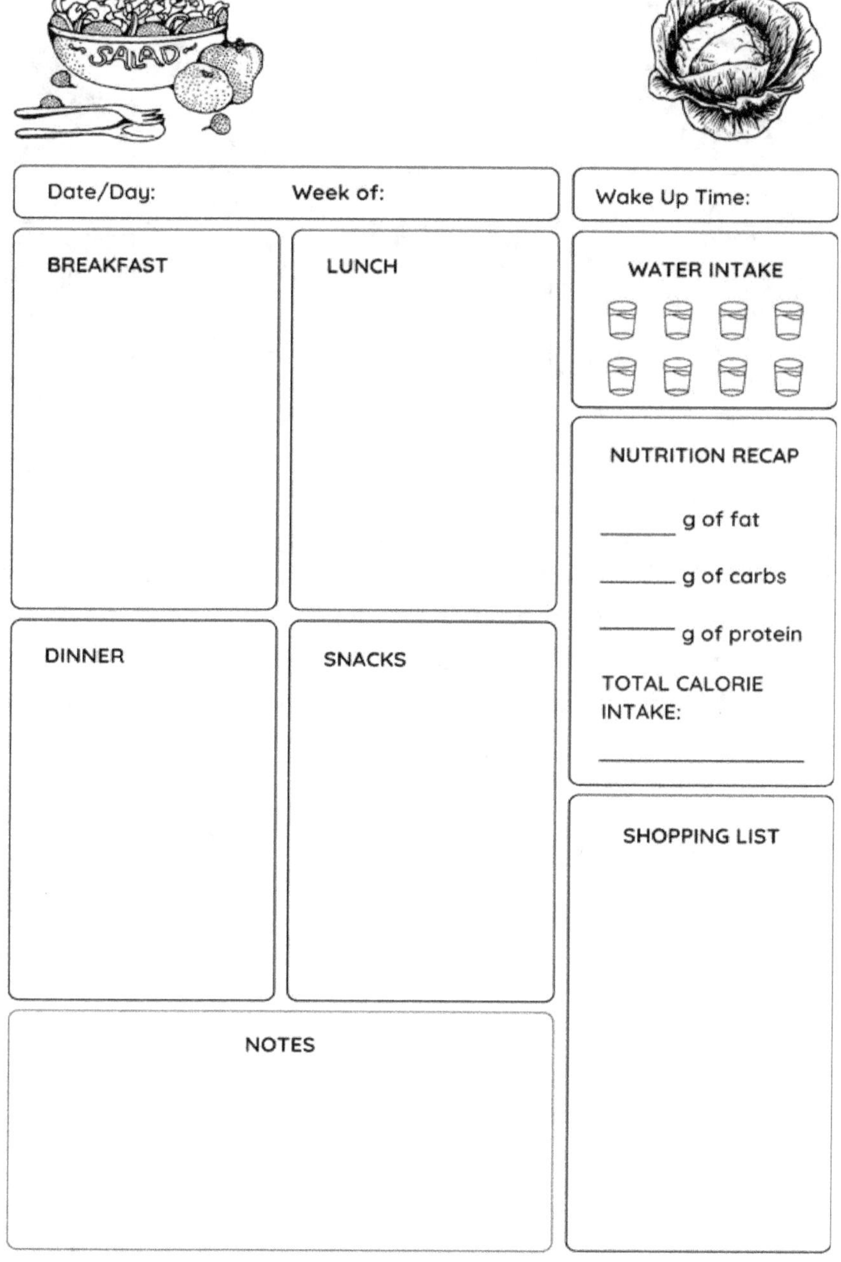

Date/Day:	Week of:		Wake Up Time:

BREAKFAST

LUNCH

WATER INTAKE

NUTRITION RECAP

_______ g of fat

_______ g of carbs

_______ g of protein

TOTAL CALORIE INTAKE:

DINNER

SNACKS

SHOPPING LIST

NOTES

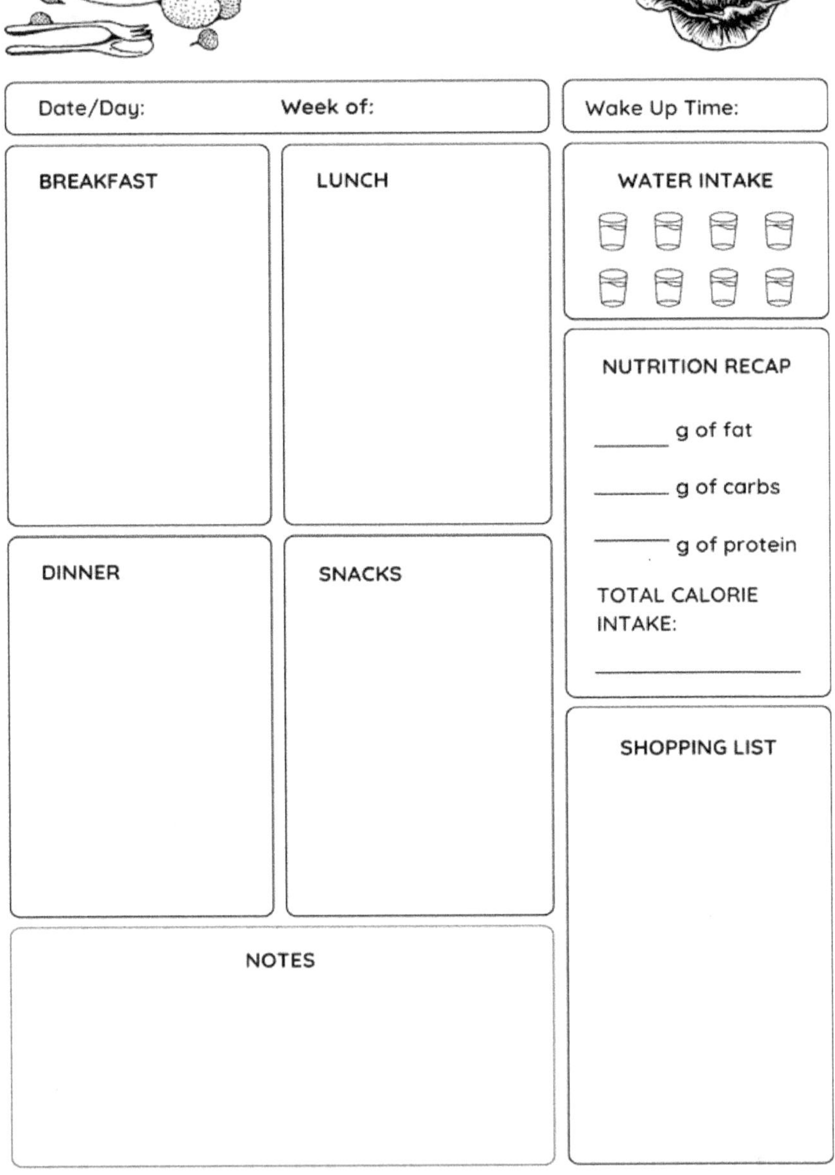

| Date/Day: | Week of: | Wake Up Time: |

BREAKFAST

LUNCH

WATER INTAKE

NUTRITION RECAP

__________ g of fat

__________ g of carbs

__________ g of protein

TOTAL CALORIE INTAKE:

____

DINNER

SNACKS

SHOPPING LIST

NOTES

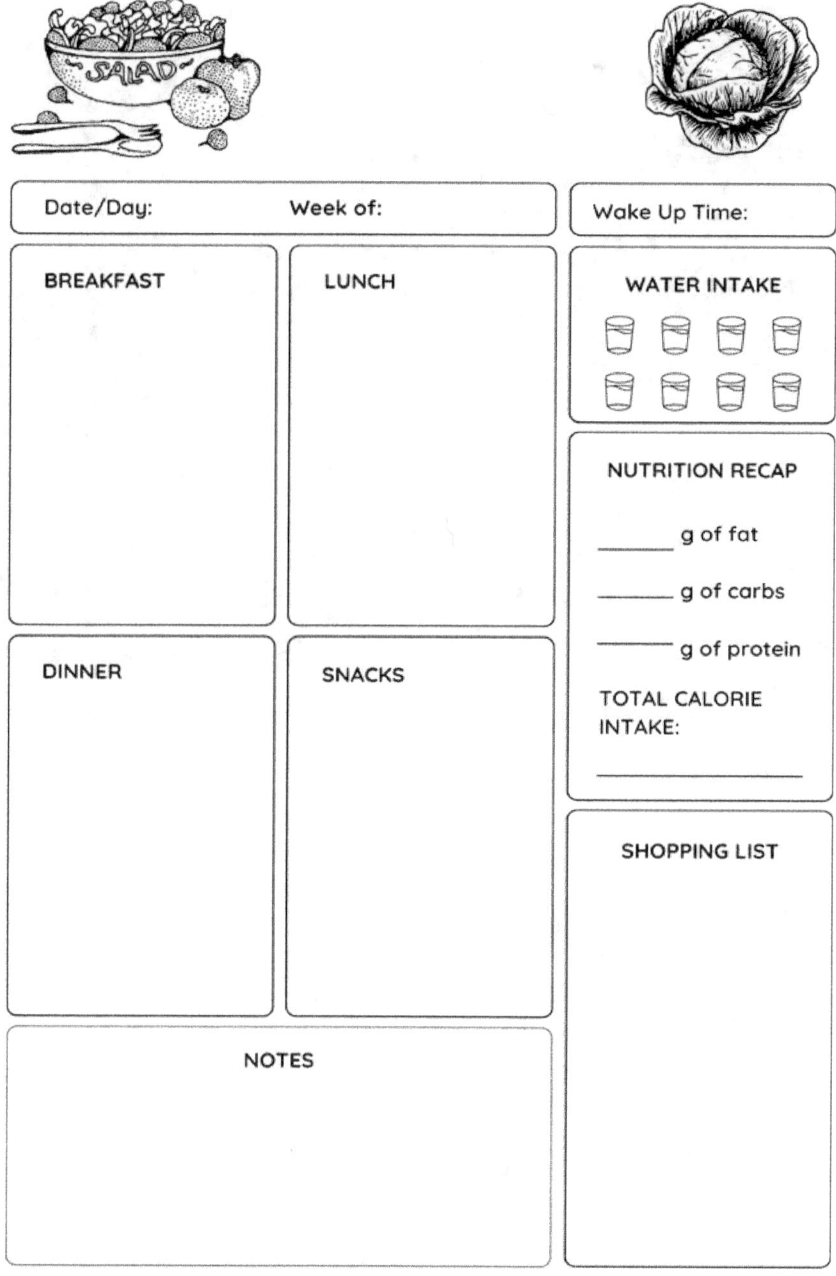

Date/Day: Week of:

Wake Up Time:

BREAKFAST

LUNCH

WATER INTAKE

NUTRITION RECAP

________ g of fat

________ g of carbs

________ g of protein

TOTAL CALORIE INTAKE:

____

DINNER

SNACKS

SHOPPING LIST

NOTES

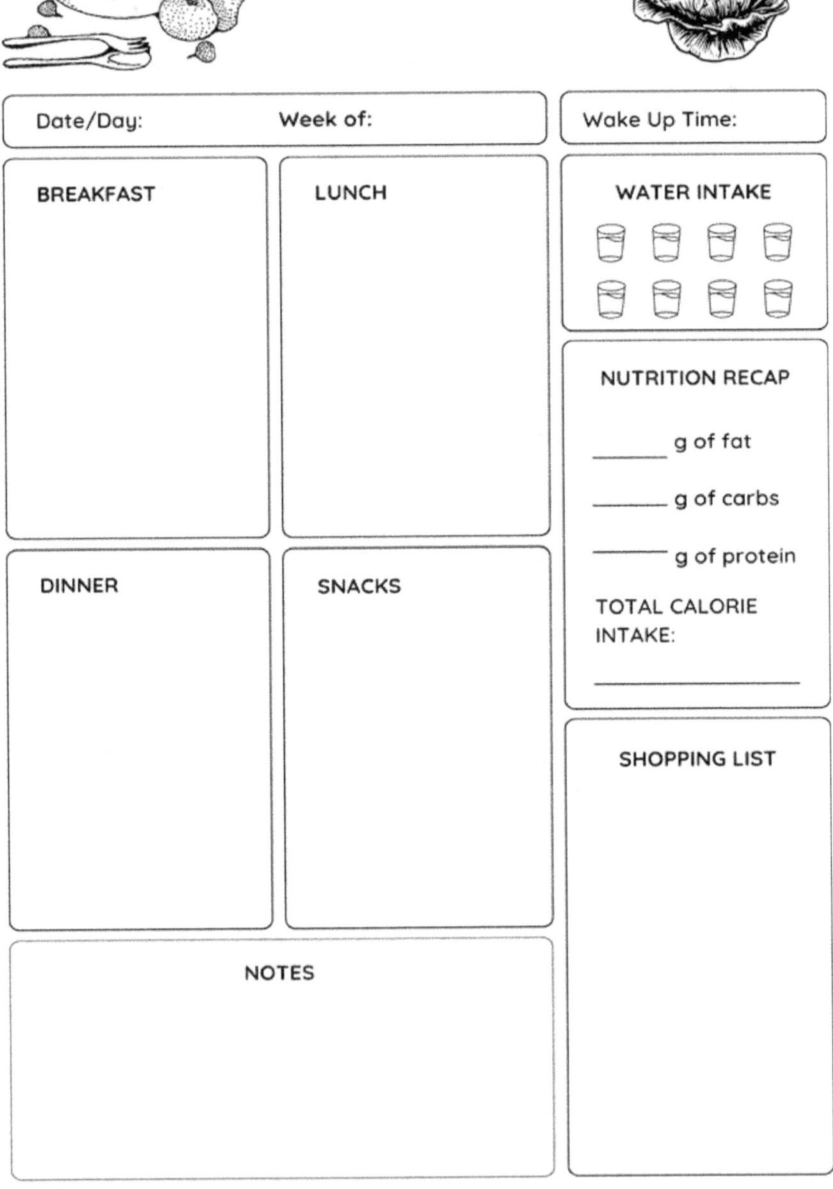

<table>
<tr><td colspan="2">Date/Day: Week of:</td><td>Wake Up Time:</td></tr>
<tr><td>**BREAKFAST**</td><td>**LUNCH**</td><td>**WATER INTAKE**</td></tr>
<tr><td>**DINNER**</td><td>**SNACKS**</td><td>**NUTRITION RECAP**

_______ g of fat

_______ g of carbs

_______ g of protein

TOTAL CALORIE INTAKE:
_______________</td></tr>
<tr><td colspan="2">**NOTES**</td><td>**SHOPPING LIST**</td></tr>
</table>

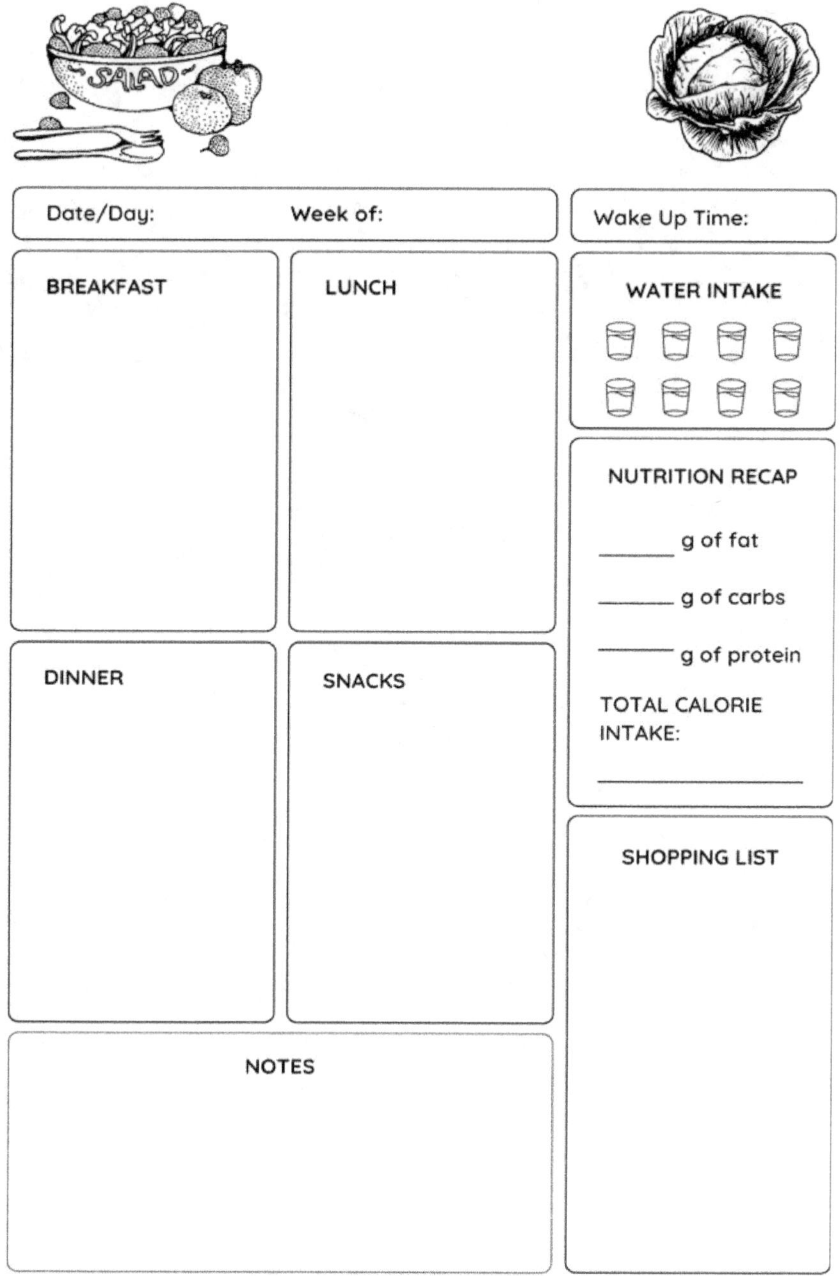

Date/Day: Week of:

Wake Up Time:

BREAKFAST

LUNCH

WATER INTAKE

NUTRITION RECAP

_________ g of fat

_________ g of carbs

_________ g of protein

TOTAL CALORIE INTAKE:

____

DINNER

SNACKS

SHOPPING LIST

NOTES